# AIDS
## Pathology, Diagnosis, Treatment & Prevention
### Third Edition

# AIDS

# Pathology, Diagnosis, Treatment & Prevention

## Third Edition

**Dr. Govind Srivastava** MD, MNAMS
Senior Dermatologist and Reader,
Skin Institute and School of Dermatology,
Greater Kailash, New Delhi
Secretary, Skin Institute Research Society, New Delhi
Editor, "Asian Clinics in Dermatology" and "Dermatology Times"
Deputy Director, Dr. Behl's Wholistic Health Centre,
Ashok Vihar, New Delhi

**Dr. Amita Srivastava** PhD
Chief, Microbiological Database, New Delhi

CBS

**CBS PUBLISHERS & DISTRIBUTORS PVT. LTD.**

NEW DELHI • BENGALURU • PUNE • KOCHI • CHENNAI

ISBN : 81-239-1420-2

**First Edition : 1994**
**Second Edition : 2003**
Reprint : 2004, 2006
**Third Edition : 2007**
Reprint : 2009, 2012



Published by Satish Kumar Jain and produced by V.K. Jain for
CBS Publishers & Distributors Pvt. Ltd.,
CBS Plaza, 4819/XI Prahlad Street, 24 Ansari Road, Daryaganj,
New Delhi - 110002, India. • Website: www.cbspd.com
e-mail: delhi@cbspd.com, cbspubs@airtelmail.in
Ph.: 23289259, 23266861, 23266867 • Fax: 011-23243014

*Branches:*

- ***Bengaluru:*** Seema House, 2975, 17th Cross, K.R. Road,
  Bansankari 2nd Stage, Bengaluru - 560070
  • Ph.: +91-80-26771678/79 • Fax: +91-80-26771680
  • E-mail: cbsbng@gmail.com, bangalore@cbspd.com
- ***Pune:*** Bhuruk Prestige, Sr. No. 52/12/2+1+3/2,
  Narhe, Haveli (Near Katraj-Dehu Road By-pass), Pune - 411041
  • Ph.: +91-20-64704058/59, 32342277 • E-mail: pune@cbspd.com
- ***Kochi:*** 36/14, Kalluvilakam, Lissie Hospital Road,
  Kochi - 682018, Kerala • Ph.: +91-484-4059061-65
  • Fax: +91-484-4059065 • E-mail: cochin@cbspd.com
- ***Chennai:*** 20, West Park Road, Shenoy Nagar, Chennai - 600030
  Ph.: +91-44-26260666, 26208620 • Fax: +91-44-42032115
  • E-mail: chennai@cbspd.com

*Printed at* :
Glorious Printers, Delhi

*Dedicated*
*To*
*The Scientists*
*Exploring Ceaselessly*
*The Therapy Of*
*This Dreaded Syndrome*
*For Over Two Decades*
*Risking Their*
*Precious Lives*
*&*
*To The Patients Who Have*
*Braved This Scourge*

# Preface to the Third Edition

Acquired immunodeficiency Syndrome (AIDS) emerged in the world at a time when the guardians of medicine were on relentless spree of wiping off dreaded diseases, and were planning to enter the 21st century with all the celebrity. This challenge, however, has been accepted with all zeal, and thousands of centres and laboratories the world over are exploring the prospects for early diagnosis, reliable treatment and eradication of AIDS from the globe. Numerous reports on various facets of AIDS have figured in several journals and the contemporary texts, eversince the first reports of the entity appeared in early 1981. Press is also giving justifiably ample coverage to it, while a worldwide surveillance is on for assessing the extent of the problem. Twenty first century has spent four years, but 'health for all" is still faraway. AIDS patients have increased at an alarming rate in the developing countries, and challenges to research workers are increasing. This pandemic is causing a dramatic and devastating impact in their health care facilities. A significant yield of the advanced research in this field are numerous anti-AIDS preparation which are increasingly used to curtail is progress and improve quality of life of these patients. Anti-AIDS vaccines are in an advanced stage of trials, infusing hope for an AIDS cure. The present manuscript updates the latest developments in this field, and gives a concise information on the subject both for medical and non-medical persons dealing with such patients.

GOVIND SRIVASTAVA M.D. MNAMS
AMITA SRIVASTAVA Ph.D

# Preface to the Third Edition

# Contents

| | | Page No. |
|---|---|---|
| | *Preface* | vii |
| 1. | History Repeats Itself | 1 |
| 2. | AIDS – The 'Invisible' Inferno | 16 |
| 3. | The Human Immunodeficiency Virus (HIV-1) | 28 |
| 4. | The Clinical Features | 37 |
| 5. | Pediatric AIDS | 46 |
| 6. | Pathology of AIDS | 57 |
| 7. | Spectrum of Infections | 74 |
| 8. | Cancers – The Added Agony | 95 |
| 9. | AIDS-Related Complex (ARC) – An Early Clue | 101 |
| 10. | Diagnostic Approach | 105 |
| 11. | Treatment | 115 |
| 12. | Prevention – Only Sure Cure | 139 |
| 13. | Afterthought | 149 |
| 14. | Appendices | |
| | *Appendix I* *AIDS/HIV Worldwide* | 152 |
| | *Appendix II* *Incidence of AIDS in the United States* | 157 |
| | *Appendix III* *Patients classified through mode of transmission and age group in USA* | 158 |
| | *Appendix IV* *Twenty Queries & their Answers* | 159 |
| | *Appendix V* *Significance of a Laboratory Test* | 167 |
| | *Appendix VI* *NACO: State AIDS Control Socieities* | 168 |
| | *Appendix VII* *Can this be AIDS?* | 171 |
| *Bibliography* | | 187 |
| *Index* | | 201 |

# Contents

# 1

# History Repeats Itself

From the times immemorial, man has been a victim of lethal infectious disorders, the infecting agents varying from period to period. In the past, there used to be outbreaks of dreaded diseases that, assumed gigantic epidemic proportion in a short time, and took a heavy toll of human life. By the middle of the twentieth century, the ever-widening scientific horizon had successfully checked many such epidemics, and developed numerous medicines and vaccines to curtail the rest. Nevertheless, as we were heading towards a more healthy and vigorous 21st century, our expectations met a serious setback in the form of the emergence of the most invincible plague, AIDS – the Acquired Immune Deficiency Syndrome, in early months of the year 1981. By this time, man had apparently conquered all the major facets of Nature, when the Nature challenged him with this hitherto novel yet fatal illness.

## HISTORICAL

The discovery of Acquired immune deficiency syndrome was based on the strong suspicion, as lots of unusual infections and Kaposi's sarcoma were recorded in a short course of time. In May 1981, *Pneumocystis carinii* pneumonia and other opportunistic infections, as well as Kaposi's sarcoma cases were discovered by the Centres for Disease Control, in previously healthy young homosexual men in scintillating cities, New York and San Francisco. Such infections could only be anticipated in severely immunocompromised host, and their occurrence in these apparently healthy men baffled the experts. Thus, it suggested an idiopathic, acquired abnormality of the immune system. Simultaneously, unprecedented occurrence of Kaposi's sarcoma in the North America was equally intriguing, and acted as an additional pointer towards this strange immunodeficiency. Numerous theories were propounded for this phenomenon, but none could explain it satisfactorily. In the following months, as the surveillance for this mysterious illness was in progress by the Centres for Disease Control (CDC) task force, it was noticed that several heterosexual intravenous drug abusers as well as heterosexual haemophiliac patients also had developed similar disorders. It also came to light that no patient with such confusing illness (fitting the definition of AIDS by the Task Force) was found prior to the year 1978, thus making this syndrome a new entity, and not an old, hitherto undiscovered disease. Its occurrence in males with various sexual habits and/or numerous partners suggested a transmissible agent capable of mediating an immunosuppressive state, being perpetuated from person to person by body fluids. In haemophiliacs, however, the transmission appeared to be mediated via infected blood products, and possibly infected apparatus and/or needles, the latter strongly incriminated in intravenous drug-abusers. These circumstantial evidences stressed beyond doubt that AIDS is caused by an infectious agent. The Centres for Disease Control, thus, redefined AIDS for the purpose of surveillance and reporting. It included (a) young adult patient developing a reliably diagnosed disease such a *P. carinii* pneumonia or *Kaposi's sarcoma*, suggesting an underlying immune defect, and (b) this occurred in the absence of cellular immune deficiency ascribed to other factors.

A human T-lymphotrophic retrovirus was the most likely cause of AIDS, prompting many investigators to explore this crucial aspect. The virus was isolated, nevertheless with great difficulty, and was initially designated as *Lymphadenopathy Associated Virus* (LAV), as it was isolated from a patient with *Lymph Adenopathy Syndrome* (LAS). However, a detailed analysis of these isolated viral particles could, unfortunately, not be undertaken, as it was cultivated only in limited amount, and thus its association with AIDS could not be ascertained. Nonetheless, evidence favouring such a human T-lymphotrophic retrovirus as the etiologic agent of AIDS continued to accumulate. They included (a) the prevalence of HTLV-I alongwith AIDS, (b) the precedent in cats for a retrovirus (feline leukaemia virus) causing both target cell proliferation and depletion, (c) the significantly higher incidence of the presence of serum antibodies that reacted with antigens present on HTLV-I infected cells, and (d) a higher prevalence of antibodies to HTLV-I envelop proteins in the AIDS patients. However, a lower frequency of antibodies to HTLV-I core proteins stressed that this retro-virus of AIDS was only distantly related to the former.

A major breakthrough was achieved in the year 1983, when this virus was successfully transmitted to subclones of human T-cell line without death of the latter, thus, making its biochemical and immunologic identification possible. It was then designated as human T-cell leukaemia (lymphotrophic) virus type III (HTLV-III). Later, The International Committee on Viral Nomenclature declared that this virus shall henceforth be known as Human Immuno-deficiency Virus type-I (HIV-1).

Prior to the discovery of this virus, the incubation period of AIDS was considered to range from 15 to 18 months. However, in infants, the disease often appeared by 8th month of age. While, in cases with blood transfusion, it averaged over 24 months. The present evidence suggests that the cumulative incidence (attack rate) of AIDS in HIV-I seropositive cases usually varies from 4 to 19 per cent annually during the 3rd and 4th seropositive year. Thereafter, it is likely to decline. At five years after seroconversion, roughly 7 per cent of homosexuals develop AIDS, while 25 per cent demonstrate persistent generalised lymphadenopathy. However, a majority of patients belonging to the latter category do not convert to full-blown AIDS.

## Magnitude of Global Problem

According to the *Joint United Nations Programme on HIV/AIDS*, as of the end of the year 2001, the following trends of the worldwide epidemic (or pandemic) of HIV are evident:

(i) Till date, 40 million people are estimated to be living with HIV/AIDS. Of these, 37.2 million are adults, 17.6 million are women, and 2.7 million are children under 15.

(ii) During 2001, AIDS caused the deaths of an estimated 3 million people, including 1.1 million women and 580,000 children under 15.

(iii) Women are becoming increasingly affected by HIV. Approximately 48%, or 17.6 million, of the 37.2 million adults living with HIV or AIDS worldwide are women.

(iv) The overwhelming majority of people with HIV-approximately 95% of the global total-now live in the developing world.

At the turn of the new century, the breakup of the patients is briefed in the figure 1.1, when patients living with HIV/AIDS were estimated to be 36.1 million. Geographic area/country-wise details have been given in the Appendix I.

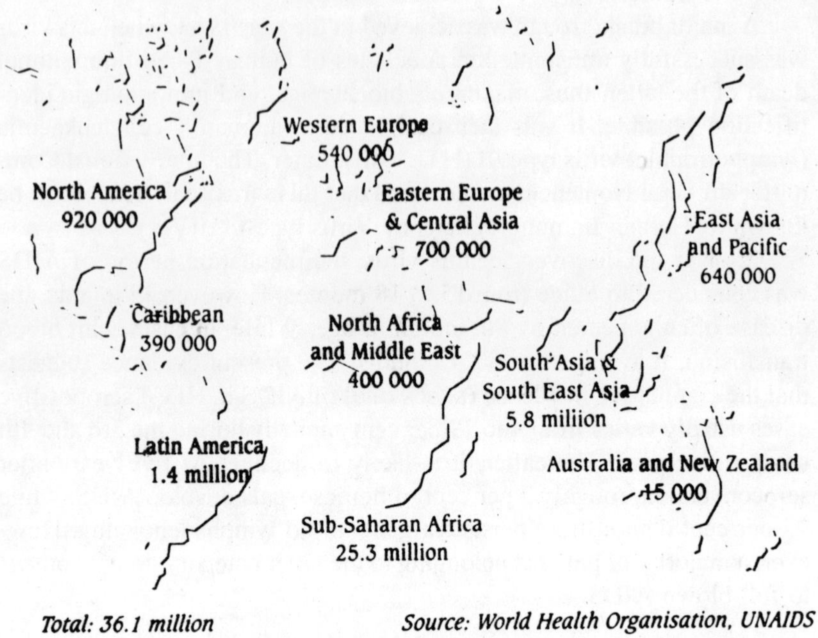


**Fig. 1. The number of adults and children estimated to be living with HIV/AIDS at the end of 2000.**

In the developed countries, despite the current low prevalence of maternal and paediatric HIV infection, AIDS has become an important cause of death in women and children. In the US, AIDS ranked as a leading cause of death in women of child-bearing age and tenth leading case of death in children between 1-4 years. Because of lack of reliable cause-and age-specific mortality rates, it is difficult to compute similar figures in the developing countries. Prior to the advent of AIDS, UN had projected that the under 5 mortality rate would decline from 164/1000 live births in 1988 to 130/1000 by 2000 AD. Current estimates indicate that under 5 year mortality was 166/1000 in 1988 and is likely to rise to 185/1000 by 2000 AD. A similar trend is likely to be seen in the maternal and adult mortality rates too. HIV has thus wiped out the decline in mortality rates achieved by the three decades of toil.

## DEMOGRAPHY

### India

India has the unique distinction of being the first country in the world to initiate a systematic nationwide serosurveillance among asymptomatic men and women belonging to high- and low-risk groups, to obtain information on the magnitude and the major mode of transmission of HIV infection, much before the AIDS case were reported from the country. In 1986, Indian Council of Medical Research organised the national serosurveillance for HIV infection. Heterosexual promiscuity was found to be the major mode of transmission of HIV infection in India. However, it became obvious that the infection is not confined to promiscuous men and women. HIV infection was also detected among 'general population': blood donors, spouses of promiscuous persons, children born to seropositive women and persons receiving blood/blood product infusion. Serourvey showed that HIV infection is present both in urban and rural areas.

The latest data recorded by NACO on HIV/AIDS surveillance as an May 31, 2005, shows a total of 1,09,349 AIDS patients, of which 77,457 are males and 31,892 are females. The risk/transmission categories are enumerated in the table 1.1, while age and sex distribution is depicted in the table 1.2. Compared to the world statistics on women – AIDS patients, where around 48 per cent are women, the male: female ratio in India is around 2.5 : 1.

**Table 1.1: Risk Transmission Categories**

| Categories | No. of cases | Percentage |
|---|---|---|
| Sexual | 93964 | 85.93 |
| Perinatal transmission | 3957 | 3.61 |
| Blood and blood products | 2201 | 2.01 |
| Injectable Drug Users | 2661 | 2.43 |
| History not available | 6566 | 6.02 |
| Total | 109349 | 100.00 |

**Table 1.2: Age and Sex distribution**

| Age group | Male | Female | Total |
|---|---|---|---|
| 0-14 yrs. | 2799 | 1945 | 4744 |
| 15-29 yrs. | 21440 | 14149 | 35589 |
| 30-44 yrs. | 47312 | 14159 | 61471 |
| > 45 yrs. | 5906 | 1639 | 7545 |
| Total | 77457 | 31892 | 109349 |

**Table 1.3: Statewise breakup of AIDS patients included (NACO)**

| S. No. | State/UT | AIDS Cases |
|---|---|---|
| 1 | Andhra Pradesh | 11819 |
| 2 | Assam | 225 |
| 3 | Arunachal Pradesh | 0 |
| 4 | A & N Islands | 33 |
| 5 | Bihar | 155 |
| 6 | Chandigarh (UT) | 1181 |
| 7 | Delhi | 950 |
| 8 | Daman & Diu | 1 |
| 9 | Dadra & Nagar Haveli | 0 |
| 10 | Goa | 555 |
| 11 | Gujarat | 5561 |
| 12 | Haryana | 469 |
| 13 | Himachal Pradesh | 239 |
| 14 | Jammu & Kashmir | 2 |
| 15 | Karnataka | 2478 |
| 16 | Kerala | 1769 |
| 17 | Lakshadweep | 0 |
| 18 | Madhya Pradesh | 1347 |
| 19 | Maharashtra | 13402 |
| 20 | Orissa | 128 |
| 21 | Nagaland | 736 |
| 22 | Manipur | 2866 |
| 23 | Mizoram | 106 |
| 24 | Meghalaya | 8 |
| 25 | Pondicherry | 302 |
| 26 | Punjab | 292 |
| 27 | Rajasthan | 1153 |
| 28 | Sikkim | 8 |
| 29 | Tamilnadu | 52036 |
| 30 | Tripura | 5 |
| 31 | Uttar Pradesh | 1383 |
| 32 | West Bengal | 2397 |
| 33 | A.bad Mun. Corp. | 520 |
| 34 | Mumbai M.C | 7223 |
| | Total | 109349 |

The highest number of the AIDS patients have been recorded in Tamil Nadu (52,036), followed by Maharashtra (13,402) (Table 1.3). In India, around 80% of cases are due to heterosexual transmission against the world statistics of about 60%. Blood and blood product transfusion is responsible for about 16% of cases, while the global figure is 3%. Drug addicts constitute about 4% of cases. HIV-positive cases are increasing in alarming proportions among high-risk groups like prostitutes and drug abusers. In the United States and Africa, homosexuals from a very important high risk group. So far in India, this does not appear to be a significant factor. However, many cases may be under-reported.

## HIV Estimates for year 2001

(based on HIV Sentinel surveillance round-2001, NACO)

The estimates for 1998, 1999 and 2000 were 3.5 million infections, 3.7 million infections and 3.86 million infections respectively. The number of new infections can therefore be put at 0.11 million (3.97-3.86) in 2001 as compared to 0.16 million (3.86-3.7) in 2000. This shows that while the epidemic still spreading in the country, there is a gradual decrease in new infections. Over a period of time, the new infections may reduce to a negligible number, which is an indicator of the plateauing of the epidemic. The existing indicators shows that such a phenomena may occur in next 3-4 year if a strong and effective programme is implemented in all the States/Union territories. This also indicates that in the north region of the country where the epidemic is still at low level, the focus should be to maintain its *status quo*. (NACO, 2002)

## HIV Sentinel Surveillance Round: 2001 (NACO)

HIV Sentinel surveillance system has proved to be the best system to monitor trends of HIV infection in specific high-risk groups as well as low risk groups. Few selected sentinel sites representing the various groups of population would be screened for HIV prevalence and its trends are monitored over a period of time. Accordingly, the Sentinel surveillance for HIV infection was taken up in 55 sentinel sites in 1994, which was expanded, to 180 Sentinel Sites in 1998 in various parts of the country. During year 2000, the round was conducted in 232 sentinel sites in various risk groups. The population groups and sites are chosen based on information of risk behaviour of various risk groups for HIV infection. The high-risk groups of population include patients attending STD clinics, MSM and Intravenous drug users while low risk of population includes mothers attending antenatal clinics (ANC). Based on consistent high prevalence of HIV as shown by HIV sentinel data of last three rounds, 49 districts have been identified as high prevalence districts (Table 1.4).

**Table 1.4: Districts with high prevalence of HIV among STD, IDU and ANC attendees: Statewise 2001 (NACO, 2002)**

| S. No. | Name of State/UT | Name of the district | |
|---|---|---|---|
| 1. | Andhra Pradesh (7) | Hyderabad | Chittoor |
| | | Vishakhapatnam | Kurnool |
| | | Guntur | Warrangal |
| | | East Godavari | |
| 2. | Goa (1) | South-Goa | |
| 3. | Gujarat (3) | Ahmedabad | Baroda |
| | | Surat | |
| 4. | Karnataka (10) | Bangalore | Dakshin Kannada |
| | | Mysore | (Mangalore) |
| | | Dharwad (Hubli) | Udipi |
| | | Bellary | Bijapur |
| | | Belgaum | Shyamraj Nagar |
| | | Gulbarga | (Kollegal) |
| 5. | Maharashtra (14) | Nagpur | Kolhapur |
| | | Sangli | Nasik |
| | | Pune | Satara |
| | | Aurangabad | Solapur |
| | | Chandrapur | Thane |
| | | Latur | Mumbai |
| | | Ratnagiri | Jalgaon |
| 6. | Manipur (4) | Imphal | Bishnupur |
| | | Churachandpur | Thoubal |
| 7. | Nagaland (3) | Kohima | Mokok Chung |
| | | Tuensang | |
| 8. | Tamil Nadu (7) | Madurai | Namakkal |
| | | Trichy | Tirunelveli |
| | | Salem | Chennai |
| | | Coimbatore | |

As the HIV problem intensifies, the issues of care support for affected individuals, and prevention of HIV transmission become even more critical. Voluntary counselling and testing (VCT) is a key entry point for interventions in HIV prevention. It provides people with an opportunity to learn and accept their HIV serostatus in a confidential and enabling environment, and to cope with the stress arising out of HIV infection. VCT is an integral part of HIV prevention programs, as it is a relatively cost-effective intervention in preventing HIV transmission. Its potential benefit include:

- Earlier access to care and treatment
- Providing factual information about HIV/AIDS and clearing misconcepts
- Reduction of fear and stigma through counselling
- Creating enabling environment
- Emotional Support
- Better ability to cope with HIV related anxiety
- Improved Health status through good nutritional advice
- Motivation to initiate or maintain safer sexual practices and behaviour change
- Prevention of HIV related illness
- Motivation for drug related behaviour
- Safer blood donation
- Motivating HIV infected person to involve spouse/partner for future spread and care

Keeping in the view the importance of VCT in Prevention and Care of HIV/AIDS, NACO has decided to expand this facility up to district hospitals throughout the country. So far more than 540 VCTCs have been established in various states/UTs, which are located in medical college hospital & district hospitals.

## The United States

Although this notorious immune deficiency possibly originated in the United States, yet the onus of unfolding diverse aspects of AIDS in such a lucid and detailed way in a record short time also goes to the scientists here. It would have taken long way in finding the etiology of this mysterious disease, had it initially emerged in the developing countries, and thus it would have taken a far extensive toll of the valuable human life, and spread more relentlessly, engulfing diverse populations. Of all the AIDS patients, homosexual/bisexual males distinctly head the table. This is followed by the intravenous drug abusers. Haitians, patients receiving blood component transfusions, haemophiliacs, heterosexual contacts and children, in that order. Some AIDS patients may not fall in any of the above high-risk groups. Haitians, in particular, show a higher incidence of AIDS. Centres for Disease Control tabulations, however, use a hierarchical classifications system for risk-group assignment. Thus, patients with multiple risk-groups are assigned arbitrarily to the group that appears first on the list. And so, parental drug abusers group exclude those who are also male homosexuals, and Haitians exclude homosexuals and drug abusers, and so forth.

**Table 1.5: Age at diagnosis of AIDS patients (CDC, 2001)**

| Age group | Number of cumulative AIDS Cases |
|---|---|
| Under 5: | 6,928 |
| 5 to 12: | 2,066 |
| 13 to 19: | 4,219 |
| 20 to 24: | 27,880 |
| 25 to 29: | 103,085 |
| 30 to 34: | 175,343 |
| 35 to 39: | 177,759 |
| 40 to 44: | 131,718 |
| 45 to 49: | 77,152 |
| 50 to 54: | 40,972 |
| 55 to 59: | 22,423 |
| 60 to 64: | 12,415 |
| 65 or older: | 11,065 |

The cumulative number of AIDS cases reported to CDC in 793,026. Adult and adolescent AIDS cases total 784,032 with 649,136 cases in males and 134,845 cases in females. Through the same time period, 8,994 AIDS cases were reported in children under age 13. Total deaths of persons reported with AIDS are 457,667, including 452,111 adults and adolescents, and 5,168 children under age 15, and 388 persons whose age at death is unknown. Age distribution (age at the time of diagnosis) of AIDS patients has been recorded in the table 1.5, while race/ethnicity is given in Table 1.6.

The distribution of reported AIDS cases amongst adults and adolescent by exposure category as well as sex (if applicable) are given in the table 1.7, while the same for children (under age of 13 at the time of diagnosis) is given in the table 1.8.

**Table 1.6: Race/Ethnicity of AIDS patients in the United States (CDC, 2001)**

| Race or Ethnicity | Cumulative AIDS Cases |
|---|---|
| White, not Hispanic | 337,035 |
| Black, not Hispanic | 301,784 |
| Hispanic | 145,220 |
| Asian/Pacific Islander | 5,922 |
| American Indian/Alaska Native | 2,433 |
| Race/ethnicity unknown | 632 |

**Table 1.7: Distribution of AIDS cases according to exposure category in adults/adolescents (CDC, 2001)**

| Exposure Category | Male | Female | Total* |
|---|---|---|---|
| Men who have sex with men | 361,867 | – | 361,867 |
| Injecting Drug Use | 142,888 | 54,203 | 197,091 |
| Men who have sex with men and inject drugs | 50,066 | – | 50,066 |
| Hemophilia/coagulation disorder | 4,949 | 285 | 5,234 |
| Heterosexual contact | 30,956 | 54,782 | 85,738 |
| Recipient of blood transfusion, blood components, or tissue | 5,031 | 3,863 | 8,894 |
| Risk not reported or identified | 53,429 | 21,712 | 75,142 |

* Includes 3 persons whose sex is unknown.

**Table 1.8: Distribution of AIDS cases according to exposure categories in children (CDC, 2001)**

| Exposure Category | # of AIDS Cases |
|---|---|
| Hemophilia/coagulation disorder | 237 |
| Mother with or at risk for HIV infection | 8,207 |
| Recipient of blood transfusion, blood components, or tissue | 382 |
| Risk not reported or identified | 168 |

New York tops the 10 leading states or territories reporting the highest number of cumulative AIDS cases amongst the residents followed by California, as per statistics of Centres for Disease control-2001 survey, (Table 1.9).

**Table 1.9: Ten leading states/territories of the USA recording highest number of cumulative AIDS patients among residents**

| State/Territory | Cumulative AIDS Cases |
|---|---|
| New York | 144,106 |
| California | 121,831 |
| Florida | 83,005 |
| Texas | 55,292 |
| New Jersey | 43,017 |
| Illinois | 25,665 |
| Puerto Rico | 25,459 |
| Pennsylvania | 25,264 |
| Georgia | 23,575 |
| Maryland | 22,432 |

In many large cities in Australia, North America, and Western Europe, AIDS has become a major cause of death for young adults aged 20-40 years. During the 1990s, HIV-related disease will be among the leading causes, if not the leading cause, of death in this age group. As early as 1988, AIDS became the leading cause of death for both men and women aged 25-34 in New York City. (See also Appendix II & III).

In the chief manifestations, Kaposi's sarcoma without *Pneumocystis carinii* infection tops the list. The concomitant existence of the preceding disorders is next common, followed by other opportunistic infections. Over 90 per cent of Kaposi's sarcoma cases have been found to be belonging to homosexual AIDS group. The AIDS death in the United States have been quite high, of which patients with only Kaposi's sarcoma had a much lower mortality (29%) when compared with those with an opportunistic infection (52%). The statistics reveal that nearly 50 per cent of AIDS patients can be expected to die within 18 months of diagnosis, and some 86 per cent within 36 months of diagnosis. The prognosis of Kaposi's sarcoma alone, as mentioned *vide supra*, is however, slightly better.

## Haiti

All evidences reveal that AIDS is a new disease occurring in Haiti. Here, no Kaposi's sarcoma case was found from the year 1968 till 1983, except for an isolated case, a 54-year-old man in the year 1972. Another biopsy-proved toxoplasmosis of the central nervous system was recorded in a previously healthy 20-year-old man in 1978. Both of them, well, might be the earliest recognised AIDS victims. In the later years, however, the Haitian study group has diagnosed numerous AIDS patients. The risk-factors involved are the same as operating in the United States. Neverthe-less, they are recognised in less than 12 per cent cases. Many patients have died prior to the identification of these risk factors. Male and female prostitution acts as a chief risk-factors. A large majority (82%) belongs to the age group 20-40 years.

The chief infections recorded in AIDS patients here are tuberculosis, and severe gastrointestinal infections primarily caused by *Candida sp.* and cryptosporidiosis. Kaposi's sarcoma is the principle malignancy observed.

## Rest of the World

In the United Kingdom, over 16,000 HIV AIDS patients have been identified. The main high-incidence group recognised in Europe are the persons from Central Africa. In Europe too, many AIDS -victims do not reveal identified risk factors. On the whole, homosexual men account for nearly 3/4th of AIDS patients with identified risk factors. Homosexuals are followed by haemophiliacs and not parental drug abusers, a finding in contrast to that seen in the United States where intravenous drug abusers outnumber haemophiliacs. Parental drug abusers account for a relatively low proportion of AIDS in Europe.

In Central Africa, the epidemic probably began as early as 1950. The main modes of spread are heterosexual and maternofetal, the highest infection rates being seen in urban area (10-20% of the general urban population in some estimates) and especially in prostitutes, among whom in Nairobi the rate of HIV seropositively rose from 4% in 1981 to 61% in 1985. Taking into account extensive underdiagnosis, under-reporting, and reporting delays, WHO estimates that by 1992 close to 1 million adult AIDS cases had already occurred in sub-Saharan Africa.

In Africa, the epidemiological factors closely resemble those seen in Haiti. The chief complaints of these patients include fever (89%), diar-rhoea (80%), severe weight loss (98%) and oral/oesophageal candidiasis (71%). Persistent generalised lymphadenopathy (PGL) is observed in roughly 62 per cent of them. Kaposi's sarcoma (16%), chronic mucocutaneous herpes simplex (22%) and cryptococcal meningitis (13%) occur with relatively low frequency. Heterosexual promiscuity is single gigantic factor, as majority of the AIDS patients of Central Africa reveal history of numerous female sexual partners.

The epidemiological pattern in Latin America has evolved rapidly, and in addition to the groups of HIV-infected homosexual or bisexual men. there is increasing heterosexual transmission. HIV transmission among injecting drug users also appears to be a growing problem in some countries. 20% or more of injecting drug users in some areas of Argentina, Brazil, and Uruguay have been found to be infected with HIV (See also Appendix I).

In South-East Asia, HIV transmission was initially predominant among injecting drug users, with HIV prevalence rates in certain groups of about 50% in Bangkok, Thailand, and 30% in Yangon, Myanmar. Prevalence rates of at least 10% have also been noted in a few studies in neighbouring regions. However, heterosexual transmission has been increasing rapidly among persons with multiple sex partners, and since 1989 this appears to be the predominant mode of transmission of HIV.

Several malignancies, besides Kaposi's sarcoma, have been noticed in AIDS patients. They include non-Hodgkin's lymphomas, Hodgkin's disease, chronic lymphocytic leukaemia, Burkitt's lymphoma, adenosquamous carcinoma of the lung, hepatocellular carcinoma, and carcinoma of the oropharynx. Homosexual men, in addition, have an increased risk of carcinoma of the anal canal, although unassociated with AIDS. The SEER system (population-based Surveillance, Epidemiology and End Result cancer registries) has been able to detect a grossly significant increase in these hitherto rare malignancies. Kaposi's sarcoma among never-married men, for example, showed a 50 fold increase in the San Francisco registry.

The Global Programme on AIDS (GPA) of the World Health Organisation has developed as AIDS projection model which relies on available HIV seroprevalence data and on the annual rate of progression from HIV infection to AIDS for use in areas where reporting of AIDS cases is incomplete, and where scant data are available to quantify biological and human behavioural variables. Virtually all models, including the WHO model, have projected large increases in the number of AIDS cases by the early 1990s. Such short-term projections are considered relatively reliable since most of the new AIDS cases will develop in persons already infected with HIV. Longer-term prediction is less reliable because HIV prevalence and future trends are determined by many variables, most of which are still not well understood. WHO has applied the Delphi method to project HIV prevalence from the year 1988 to mid-2000, to improve the quality of the judgements and estimates for relatively uncertain issues by the systematic use of knowledgeable "experts".

The mean value of the Delphi projection for HIV prevalence in the year 2000 is between 3 and 4 times the 1988 base estimate of 5.1 million; these projections have been used to obtain annual estimates of adult AIDS cases up to the year 2000. Coordinated HIV/AIDS prevention and control programmes are considered by the Delphi participants to be potentially capable of preventing almost half of the new HIV infections that would otherwise occur between 1988 and the year 2000. However, more than half of the approximately 5 million AIDS cases which are projected for the next decade will occur despite the most rigorous and effective HIV/AIDS prevention efforts since these AIDS cases will develop in persons whose HIV infection was acquired prior to 1989.

The long term consequences of AIDS and AIDS-related complex can only be experienced as further time elapses. The various-faceted statistical studies are yet not complete, and further serious outcome may come forward. A long term sequelae of HIV-1 may be a T-cell malignancy. Thus, the emergence of AIDS might be indicative of a major pandemic, the full extent of which at present, to our utter horror, can only be speculative. These apprehensions justify the quantum of fear, and the resultant mobilisation of man power, even in the countries where AIDS is unknown, to carry on a strict surveillance for curtailing and eradicating this pandemic at its offing, before it eradicates the mankind. This becomes all the more important as just the emergence of this pandemic has proved devastating, the long term sequelae may prove equally ruinous, and make mankind as extinct as the dinosaurs of the past.

# 2

# AIDS – The 'Invisible' Inferno

AIDS, as the name implies, is an peculiar acquired type of immunodeficiency, with consequential development of unusual and severe infections, and bizarre neoplasms, which occurs in healthy individuals without a known cause of immunodeficiency. The Centres for Disease Control (CDC), USA, initially outlined AIDS as the occurrence of a disease that is at least moderately predictive of a defect in cell-mediated immunity, developing in a person with no cause for diminished resistance to that disease. The diseases include Kaposi's sarcoma in patients under 60 years of age, primary lymphoma of the central nervous system, *Pneumocystis carinii* pneumonia, unusually extensive herpes simplex of over 5 weeks' duration, *Cryptosporidium* enterocolitis over 4 weeks' duration, oesophagitis due to *Candida albicans,* cytomegalovirus or herpes simplex virus, progressive multifocal leukoencephalopathy, and pneumonia, meningitis or encephalitis due to *Aspergillus, Candida albicans, Cryptococcus neoformans,* cytomegalovirus, *Nocardia, strongyloides, Toxoplasma gondii, Zygomyosis* or atypical mycobacteria. The infecting agent, of course, may vary from place to place, and so in places where AIDS in not a problem, a surveillance should be done in patients affected with other atypical microbes. However, by mere suspicion, the patient should never be labelled as AIDS and pre-AIDS. Thus, frank AIDS is only the end state of the HIV-1 infection (Table 2.1)

After the discovery of the causative agent of AIDS, the CDC redefined AIDS to exclude its diagnosis in case the tests for serum antibody to HIV-1/LAV are negative, all other types of HTLV/LAV test are negative, and the number of thymus-derived (T) helper lymphocytes are normal. On the other hand, the diagnosis should be considered confirmed if serologic/virologic tests are positive for HIV-1/LAV, even if no opportunistic infection is present.

Paediatric AIDS or AIDS in children under 13 years of age should have the following exclusions: (i) Congenital infections by *T. gondii* and herpes simplex virus in patients under one month of age, congenital cytomegalovirus infection in children under 5 months of age, (ii) primary immunodeficiency disease (severe combined immunodeficiency, DiGeorge Syndrome, Wiskott-Aldrich syndrome, ataxia telengiectasia, graft-versus host disease, neutropenia, agammaglobulinemia), and (iii) secondary immunodeficiency associated with immunosuppressive therapy, lymphoreticular malignancy or starvation.

**Table 2.1: CDC case definition of AIDS**

**INFECTIONS**

**Protozoal Infections**

*Pneumocystis carinii* pneumonia
Toxoplasmosis of brain
Cryptosporidiosis with diarrhoea of over 1 month's duration.

**Viral**

Cytomegalovirus (CMV)-retinitis, pneumonitis, colitis, or encephalitis.

**Fungal**

Candidiasis-esophageal, tracheal, bronchial or pulmonary Cryptococcus-meningitis (or other extrapulmonary site)

**Bacterial**

Mycobacterium avium intercellulare or *M. kansasii*-disseminated.

*Mycobacterium tuberculosis* (if extrapulmonary, and not confined only to lymph glands, in a patient who is HIV antibody positive) Recurrent non-typhoid *Salmonella* septicaemia (if patient is HIV antibody positive)

**TUMOURS**

Kaposi's sarcoma: any age if HIV antibody + ve (< 60 if HIV status unknown)

Primary CNS lymphoma

Non-Hodgkin's lymphoma of B cell type (only if patient is HIV antibody + ve)

HIV wasting syndrome ("slim disease") – if patient is HIV anti-body + ve.

Lymphoid interstitial pneumonia (LIP) in a child < 13 years

AIDS-related complex (ARC) has been designated to patients who show concurrence of two clinical conditions with two AIDS-type laboratory abnormalities. The clinical features include fever of over 100°F for over 3 months, over 15 pounds (or 10%) body-weight loss, lymphadenopathy for more than 3 months, duration, diarrhoea, fatigue and night sweats. The laboratory abnormalities include T-helper cells below 400/cumm, helper: suppressor ratio below one, elevated serum globulins, depressed blastogenesis, anergy to skin tests and leuko-thrombocytopenia.

Persistent generalised lymphadenopathy (PGL) has been observed in many persons of the high-risk groups. This can be designated to enlarged lymph nodes of the diameter 1 cm or more, occupying 2 or more non-contiguous extrainguinal sites without an identifiable etiology, and persisting for 3 months or more. The common histopathological patterns include a marked follicular hyperplasia, sometimes angioimmunoblastic lymphadenopathy pattern, and less commonly even involution. This type of lymphadenopathy, however, can easily be encountered in the developing countries including India. Thus, in these geographic area, other causes of generalised lymphadenopathy have to be diligently sought and investigated before suspecting this as a pointer for early AIDS. Naturally, AIDS-specific laboratory investigations should form a common denominator in all suspected cases of AIDS.

Simian AIDS refers to a recent outbreak of highly lethal opportunistic infections, with PGL, and laboratory abnormalities in rhesus monkeys (*Macaca mulatta*) at the Primate Research Centre in Davis, California. This, nonetheless, should not be confused with the chimpanzee model of AIDS, where the HIV-I infection is introduced by intravenous injections of a large volume of cell-free plasma of AIDS patients with HIV-I antibodies. The simian AIDS was later also seen in other species of monkeys in Southborough, Massachusettes.

Yet another term, once used to be *in vogue,* is lesser AIDS, which includes a specific group of non-life threatening clinical conditions that occur in less severe cell-mediated immune dysfunction, analogous to that seen in AIDS. Such clinical conditions include oral candidiasis, idiopathic thrombocytopenia, and herpes zoster in individuals under 60 years of age, without any known underlying reasons for their occurrence. Although natural history of lesser AIDS is ill-defined, yet it only occasionally progresses to full-blown AIDS. (See Chapter 4, Fig. 4.1)

Asymptomatic members of the high-risk group frequently show AIDS-specific subclinical immunologic abnormalities, such as low absolute number of helper/inducer cells, ratio of these cells to suppressor/cytotoxic T-lymphocytes becoming below one, unusual species of circulating, acid-labile alpha interferon, and elevated levels of $\beta_2$ microglobulin. In the developing countries where extensive and advanced investigative and diagnostic facilities are not available, the World Health Organisation has suggested a simple case definition (Table 2.2)

**Table 2.2: WHO case definition of AIDS**

**Major Signs**

1. Weight loss > 10% of body weight
2. Chronic diarrhoea > 1 month
3. Fever > 1 month (intermittent or constant)

**Minor Signs**

1. Persistent cough > 1 month
2. General pruritic dermatitis
3. Recurrent herpes zoster
4. Oropharyngeal candidiasis
5. Chronic progressive and disseminated herpes simplex infections
6. Generalised lymphadenopathy

The detailed WHO staging system for HIV infection is given in table 2.3.

**Table 2.3: WHO staging system for HIV infection and disease in adults and adolescents**

**Clinical Stage I:**

1. Asymptomatic
2. Persistent generalized lymphadenopathy (PGL)

*Performance scale 1: Asymptomatic, normal activity*

**Clinical Stage II:**

1. Weight loss < 10% of body weight
2. Minor mucocutaneous manifestations (seborrheic dermatitis, prurigo, fungal nail infections, recurrent oral ulcerations, angular cheilitis)
3. Herpes zoster, within the last 5 years
4. Recurrent upper respiratory tract infections (i.e., bacterial sinusitis)

*And/or Performance scale 2: symptomatic, normal activity*

**Clinical stage III:**

1. Weight loss, > 10% of body weight

*(Contd.)*

2. Unexplained chronic diarrhoea, > 1 month
3. Unexplained prolonged fever (intermittent or constant), > 1 month
4. Oral candidiasis (thrush)
5. Oral hairy leukoplakia
6. Pulmonary tuberculosis, within the past year
7. Severe bacterial infections (i.e., pneumonia, pyomyositis)

*And/or performance scale 3: bed-ridden, < 50% of the day during the last month*

**Clinical Stage IV:**

1. HIV wasting syndrome*
2. *Pneumocystis carinii* pneumonia
3. Toxoplasmosis of the brain
4. Cryptosporidiosis with diarrhoea, > 1 month
5. Cryptococcosis, extrapulmonary
6. *Cytomegalovirus* (CMV) disease of an organ other than liver, spleen or lymph node (ex:retinitis)
7. *Herpes simplex virus* (HSV) infection, mucocutaneous ( > 1 month) or visceral
8. Progressive multifocal leukoencephalopathy (PML)
9. Any disseminated endemic mycosis
10. Candidiasis of the oesophagus, trachea, bronchi
11. Atypical mycobacteriosis, disseminated or lungs
12. Non-typhoid *Salmonella* septicaemia
14. Lymphoma
15. Kaposi's sarcoma (KS)
16. HIV encephalopathy**

*And/or performance scale 4: bed-ridden, > 50% of the day during the last month*

---

**Note:** both definitive and presumptive diagnoses are acceptable

* Weight loss of more than 10% of body weight, plus either unexplained chronic diarrhoea ( > 1 month), or chronic weakness and unexplained prolonged fever ( > 1 month)

** Clinical findings of disabling cognitive and/or motor dysfunction interfering with activities of daily living, progressing over weeks to months, in the absence of a concurrent illness or condition other than HIV infection that could explain the findings.

## THE POPULATION GROUPS-AT-RISK

Fortunately, AIDS has almost exclusively been a disease of certain 'at risk' groups of population. This, however, does in no way render the remaining people immune or unamenable for the AIDS virus. The disease is far more prevalent in men, and over three-forth victims of AIDS are young adult males. Women, although less common victims of AIDS, are certainly at equal risk of developing the syndrome, in case they receive appropriate exposure to the virus. More so, the 'at-risk' individuals can spread the disease to their heterosexual partners, and their children. The pattern of AIDS from Haiti and Europe has revealed that the identified risk factors were however not operating in a majority of their AIDS patient. Nevertheless, it includes those persons who die before the precise history about the underlying 'at-risk' factors is extracted from them. The well-defined 'at-risk' groups are the:

(a) Homosexuals
(b) Parentral drug abusers
(c) Haitians
(d) Haemophiliacs
(e) Those receiving repeated blood product transfusions.
(f) Heterosexual partners of AIDS victims
(g) Offsprings of AIDS victims
(h) Other contacts of AIDS victims, like the laboratory technicians, doctors, and so on.

Considerable epidemiological and clinical work has been done for understanding the transmission of HIV from one person to another. Human travel to distant place is one single factor in transmission of the disease. Despite the prompt travel and subsequent spread of AIDS infection, a long latent period from time of infection to overt development of signs and symptoms of the disease make it difficult to find the source of infection. HIV is primarily a sexually transmissible disease. Homo-sexual, bisexual, and heterosexual transmission all can occur. Although sexual intercourse between males has remained the greatest risk for transmission in developed nations of Western Europe and the United States, heterosexual transmission is also increasing in these regions, but still remains less common than in Africa, Asia, or parts of the Caribbean. Transmission of HIV can occur from male to male, male to female, and female to male. Female to female transmission remains extremely rare. Worldwide, heterosexual transmission accounts for the majority of cases of HIV infection. The important factors that promote heterosexual transmission include:

1. More sexual partners
2. Frequent change of sexual partners
3. Unprotected sexual intercourse
4. Presence of sexually-transmitted diseases
5. Lack of male circumcision
6. Social vulnerability of women and young persons
7. Economic and political instability of the community

## Homosexual Men

Nearly 68 per cent of the AIDS patients in the United States have been found to be homosexual males. Homosexual persons are usually men engaged in various sexual practices with persons of their own sex. The homosexual activities include receptive anal intercourse (passive partner), insertive anal intercourse (active partner), receptive and insertive anilingus, receptive and insertive fellatio, receptive and insertive fisting, and nitrite inhalation. They may have multiple partners, all males. These people may be married and also carrying out heterosexual sex-practices with their wives. The epidemic of AIDS came to light when previously healthy men with homosexual habits suddenly flooded the hospitals with serious infections and Kaposi's sarcoma. Till date, they constitute a single large group at-risk for the development of this disease. Even in the absence of signs and symptoms of AIDS, these people show frequent immunologic dysfunctions suggestive of a smouldering AIDS. An alarming number (80%) of symptom-free homosexual men have demonstrated a markedly lowered $T_4/T_8$ ratio, chiefly, due to an elevated $T_8$ lymphocyte population. One-third of them display a cutaneous anergy, even in the absence of circulating $T_4$-lymphocyte reduction. In the course of weeks or months, they gradually show more subtle immunological changes and gradual conversion to full-blown syndrome. It has been shown that HIV-I seropositivity is closely associated with number of homosexual partners. The use of inhalant drugs such as amyl and butyl nitrite, which suggests more frequent receptive anal intercourse, seems a factor pointing towards an increased risk to develop the diseases. Nitrite inhalants can also increase the risk of Kaposi's sarcoma in susceptible subject. The magnitude of homosexuality in India is only speculative. It is, however, certain that unnatural sexual practices including homosexual acts are not uncommon in this subcontinent. Organised surveys are indicated to outline the prevalence of homosexuality in India and other developing countries, as this group of population, if not educated and prohibited, may be a potential offender in the emergence and perpetuation of AIDS in several relatively protected areas of the world.

### Parentral drug abusers

This group of people forms the second most common 'at-risk' population in the United States, while it is third commonest group in Europe. Intravenous drug abusers inject themselves and their friends with addicting drugs, using same needles and syringes time and again. About 8 to 12 per cent of homosexual/bisexual men are also seen to be parentral drug abusers. They use a variety of hallucinating drugs including morphine, heroin and cocaine. A few drugs, such as heroin, can alter T-lymphocyte receptors for nearly 2 weeks. However, the major risk-factor is the transmission of the HIV-1 virus because of sharing/reusing blood-contaminated needles and syringes in their 'shooting galleries.' In India too, there has been a recent spurt in the number of drug abusers especially in the teenagers, due to bad friendship, social insecurity and family discords. They are potential and prospective victims of this infection, and so should again be outlined in the developing countries.

### Haemophiliacs

The individuals suffering from haemophilia also seem to be the victims of AIDS. They form the second common 'at-risk' group in Europe, while third common group in the United States. In fact, the development of AIDS in haemophiliacs who had no apparent risk factors such as homosexuality and drug abuse, suggested that AIDS is likely to be caused by a transmissible agent analogous to hepatitis-B virus. These patients require clotting factors for their therapy, which in turn are derived from the pooled plasma of thousands of commercial donors. Inspite of all precautions, there remains a low level of hepatitis-B virus, which reflect as hepatitis-B seropositivity in all such recipients. A high prevalence of both hepatitis-B and AIDS in homosexual and intravenous drug abusers is a factor of transmitting the same in the clotting factor concentrates, if these people are blood donors. Haemophilia-A patients have a higher incidence of developing AIDS (3.9 per 1000) as compared to less severe haemophilia-B patients (0.7 per 1000). A HIV-1 seropositivity of 64 to 90 per cent is found among haemophilia-A patients receiving Factor VIII concentrates, as compared with 0 to 4 per cent seropositivity in haemophiliacs receiving Factor IX concentrates, denoting a possible differing ability to transmit HIV-1 by factor VIII and Factor IX. Abnormal immunologic profiles in asymptomatic haemophiliacs as wel. as their wives have also been recorded.

## Blood/Blood Product transfusion recipients

Analogous to clotted factor concentrates, blood and blood-products have also been incriminated in AIDS transmission, making their recipients a high-risk group. Tracing the source of blood usually reveals that the donor belongs to a known high-risk group. The recipients, who developed AIDS after such transfusions, were predominantly (60%) males, with an average age of 54 years, and had received multiple transfusions from different donors. To prevent this, a thorough screening by the blood-collection agencies will go a long way. Further, known high-risk individuals should voluntarily refrain from blood donation.

## Haitians

The persons belonging to Haiti from a single important high-risk group. AIDS has spread fairly rapidly in Haiti since 1980, and appears to be concentrated in and around the male-and female-prostitution centres. They may develop AIDS despite of no history of homosexual practice or drug abuse. However, nearly one-third of men with AIDS in Haiti were found to be bisexuals or had served as prostitutes for heterosexual tourists, Nevertheless homosexual promiscuity appears to be a major factor operating in Haiti, an one quarter of the victims are females.

## Female partners of AIDS patients

Patients suffering from or intubating AIDS are capable of transmitting the disease to their female partners, stressing that vaginal intercourse in equally efficient in transmitting AIDS. Nonsexual contacts however, do not seem to transmit AIDS, as HIV-1 antibody testing has been uniformly negative in routine household contacts, who share kitchen and bathroom facilities with high-risk persons or AIDS patients. Kissing, facilitating appropriate transfer of infected secretions, can, however, transmit AIDS. The clinical progression of HIV infection is similar in men and women.

Women infected with HIV have unique problems. Both oestrogen and progesterone affect the immune system and may influence the natural history of HIV disease. In addition, pregnancy is considered a state of physiologic immunocompromise. Although HIV infection does not appear to influence the outcome of pregnancy, pregnancy may modify the course of HIV infection. The rate of CD4 cell loss in HIV-infected pregnant women is faster than that in HIV-negative pregnant women or that in HIV-infected homosexual or haemophiliac men. Opportunistic infections can be especially fulminant during pregnancy. Because of the similarity in symptoms, diagnosis may also be delayed.

*Candida* infections of mucosal surfaces have been the earliest recognized, and *Candida* infections of the oropharynx and the oesophagus are usually associated with significant decrease in CD4 counts. Chronic, refractory vaginal candidiasis is frequently encountered in HIV-infected women with a low CD4 counts.

HIV-infected women with pelvic inflammatory disease have more tubo-ovarian abscess and require more surgical interventions than non-HIV-infected women.

Abnormal Papanicolaou smears and malignancies, especially of the uterine cervix, are being found with increased frequency in HIV-infected women. Human immunodeficiency virus disease appears to profoundly affect the frequency, severity, and the rate of progression of cervical neoplastic lesions.

## Infants and Children

Pediatric AIDS usually manifest itself between 6 to 20 months of age, in infants of AIDS parents or those of high-risk groups. Children of drug-abusing mothers are at particular risk. Further, incidence of transfusion associated AIDS has been found to be 6 times higher in transfused infants than in transfused adults.

Before the discovery of HIV, many childhood infections were acquired from infected blood or blood products, but presently as the screening is properly carried out, nearly all new childhood cases are attributable to maternofetal transmission; it is estimated that about one-third, of infants born to HIV-infected mothers will be infected. Infection is believed to occur usually transplacentally or, though unproven, at delivery.

## Other Contacts of AIDS patients

The doctors treating the AIDS patients, nurses, laboratory workers and other staff members are also dealing with a potentially infective disorder. Fortunately, non-sexual contacts of AIDS patients seldom contact the illness. Although HIV-1 can be transmitted by nonsexual personal contact, yet the routine precautions and current recommendations of handling AIDS patients and their specimens (discussed in chapter 12) appear effective in curtailing casual and nosocomial dissemination.

Around 5 to 10% of persons who develop AIDS initially report no identifiable risk factor for HIV infection. In due course, however, many of them are found to have a defined risk factor when a detailed history becomes available. The number of cases of HIV infection with no identifiable risk factor has not increased significantly over time, confirming the observation that HIV infection is not acquired through casual contact.

There are three major variables that explain the sexual transmission of HIV: (1) transmission efficiency, (2) number of sexual partners, and (3) seroprevalence (numbers of infected individuals in a population). HIV transmission through sexual exchange of semen or vaginal fluids is much less efficient than transmission of either gonorrhoea or hepatitis B virus. Usually, multiple sexual exposures are necessary to increase the likelihood for transmission of HIV from infected persons. It is estimated that gonorrhea may be transmitted in 22 to 25% of sexual encounters involving an infected individual, hepatitis B virus in 20 to 30% of encounters, and hepatitis C in 2% of sexual encounters, while HIV transmission occurs much less often-approximately 0.3% per sexual contact with an HIV-infected person. However, some persons have become HIV-infected after a single sexual contact, while other persons have remained uninfected after hundreds of contacts. Several factors can enhance the chances of the risk for HIV infection and are enumerated in table 2.4.

**Table 2.4: Factors increasing the risk for HIV infection**

| Sex | Factor (s) |
|---|---|
| Females: | – Cervical ectopia |
| | – Oral contraceptive use |
| | – Pregnancy |
| | – Menstruation |
| | – Genital ulcer disease |
| | – Use of crack cocaine with oral sex |
| Males: | – Uncircumcised penis |
| | – Genital ulcer disease |

## HIV vs STDS

The HIV epidemic has dramatically altered the field of sexually transmitted diseases (STDs). HIV infection is unique among sexually transmitted diseases because it can modify the clinical presentation and features of other STDs. Conversely, other STDs can affect the transmission of HIV. There are a variety of mechanisms by which the coexistence of other sexually transmissible diseases (STDs) may increase the infectivity of HIV. Both *Chlamydia trachomatis* and *Treponema pallidum* infection appear to increase HIV-1 replication, while *Hemophilus ducreyi* infection increases CCR5 chemokine coreceptor expression by macrophages. In men, urethritis due to *Neisseria gonorrheae* and *Trichomonas* has been shown to increase the amount of HIV-1 in semen. Likewise, in women, cervicovaginal fluids contain more HIV-1, as well as CD4 cells when additional STDs are present. *Chlamydia trachomatis, Neisseria gonorrheae,* and *Trichononas,* or diseases producing genital ulcers such as herpes simplex virus, chancroid (*Hemophilus ducreyi*) or syphilis (*Treponema pallidum*), all enhance infectivity by HIV. Treatment of these STDs may help to reduce the number of new HIV-1 cases.

The cofactor effect of genital ulcer disease is approximately five times higher for female-to-male than for male-to-female transmission. A higher prevalence of STD's in the population may further equalize HIV transmission between the sexes.

# 3

# The Human Immunodeficiency Virus (HIV-1)

The etiology of AIDS is now well established. It is caused by a retrovirus, initially named the Human T-Cell Leukaemia (lymphotropic) Virus (HTLV) number III, and designated subsequently as HIV-1. For the isolation of this virus, phytohaemagglutinin-P (mitogen) stimulated mononuclear cells prepared from peripheral blood, bone marrow and other tissues of the patients and donors have to be established in cell culture using growth medium supplemented with T-Cell growth factor. The virus is detected by (a) virus reverse transcriptase activity in the supernatant fluids, (b) transmitting virus to fresh normal human T-lymphocytes, or to established T-cell lines, (c) electron microscopic examination of fixed and sectioned cells, and (d) testing for antigen expression by indirect immunofluorescene (or Western blot procedures) using serum from the sero-positive donors. The primary cells from patients produce the virus in 2-3 weeks after introduction in tissue cultures, following which its production declines. A second production of virus occurs after several weeks of initial crop. Coincident with viral expression, there is a loss of viable cells in general, and of those helper/inducer ($OKT_4/Leu^{3a+}$) phenotype, in particular. The frequency of HIV-I isolation is maximum (80%) in ARC patients, followed by AIDS (50%) and healthy at-risk individuals (20%). An addition of antibody to alpha-interferon usually facilitate the detection of this virus, as is the addition of hydrocortisone. HIV-1 is a 100-120 nm diameter virus, produced in abundance from infected cells, by budding from the cell membrane. A characteristic cylindrical core can be identified in many presumably mature virions.

The etiologic association of this virus with AIDS can, thus, be confirmed by its isolation from the blood of AIDS patients. It is complimented by strong seroepidemiologic evidence, demonstrating antibodies to HIV-1 in the sera of over 90 per cent AIDS and ARC patients, using indirect membrane immunofluorescene, enzyme-linked immunosorbence assay (ELISA) or Western blot analysis techniques. The control sera from healthy individuals have been uniformly negative. These antibodies could, however, be demonstrated in many high-risk persons. The serum antibody to HIV-1 can be detected in majority of AIDS patients at the onset of clinical symptoms, but its titres usually fall as the disease advances. The titres are thus significantly high in ARC patients. These sero-epidemiologic investigations are indicated in screening the high-risk population as well as blood donors.

## BIOLOGIC PROPERTIES OF HIV-1

The pathologic picture observed *in vivo* due to this virus reflects, to much extent, the *in vitro* characteristics of HIV-1 infected cells, which is outlined below. Of the established cell lines, a neoplastic aneuploid T-cell line derived from an adult with lymphoid leukaemia (termed HT) has been found to be susceptible to its infection. The HT cell population has been extensively cloned to improve permissiveness for HIV-1 and to preserve permanent growth and continuous production of the virus. Cell numbers are seen to decline upto 10-90 per cent from the initial cell count, within 6 days after infection.

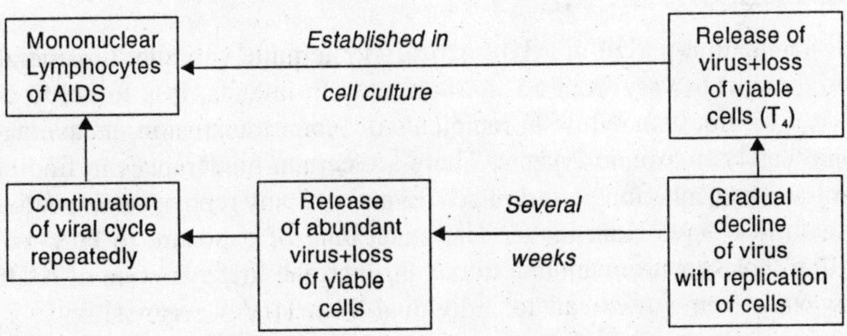


Moreover, a high proportion of multi-nucleated giant cells can be consistently observed in all infected clones. Besides HT, there are other

T or pre T-human cell lines, such as JM, CEM-CCRF, Molt-3 and RPMI 8402, which can be infected by HIV-1, and thus produce the virus. A few B-lymphoblastic lines too have this property. The common properties of HTLV viruses are summarised in Table 3.1 & 3.2.

**Table 3.1: Properties of HTLV viruses**

1. Exogenous viruses isolated from mature T-cells in general, and $OKT_4$ + cells in particular.
2. Target cells are again T-cells (*in vitro*), though may infect other cells also.
3. Possess cross-reacting antigens.
4. Have reverse transcriptase with similar properties.
5. Possess major core proteins of similar size.
6. Have pX sequence at the 3′ end of the genome.
7. Exhibit same nucleotide sequence homology under nonstringent hybridization conditions.
8. Can induce formation of multi-nucleated giant cells, by inducing T-cell fusion.

The exact pathogenesis of profound cytopathologic effect exerted by HIV-1 on infected $T_4$ cells is not known. It is believed that these infected cells liberate potent immunoregulatory factors which in turn suppress the functions of cells of immune system including T-cells, as the supernatant fluid from fresh cultures is observed to inhibit T-and B-cells activation and maturation.

## INCUBATION PERIOD

The incubation period of AIDS appears to be quite variable. In general, it is thought to vary from 15 to 28 months. In infants, it is found to be shorter (8 months). While in recipients of blood transfusion, its average value has been around 2 years. There are certain hinderances in finding the precise incubation period of AIDS, and in many reports retrospective calculations have been made. The exact date of exposure to HIV-1 is difficult to ascertain in an individual. Further, the first symptom of AIDS may vary from individual to individual-from HIV-1 seropositivity, $T_4$ cells reduction, trivial infections, generalized lymphadenopathy, Kaposi's sarcoma, to life-threatening infections.

**Table 3.2: Salient features of HIV**

1. A member of the *lentivirus* subfamily of retroviridae.
2. Genetic information is encoded in 2 RNA strands.
3. The RNA is surrounded by p18 and p24, the two protein coats.
4. It possesses a spiked envelope, whose outer portion in gp 120, while the stalk that penetrates is gp 41.
5. The 3 genes common to all retroviruses are *gag, pol* and *env. Gag* codes for p24 and p18, *Pol* codes for the enzyme reverse transcriptase and *Env* codes for the synthesis of gp 120 and gp 41.
6. It also contains non structural genes *tat, art, 3' orf. Tat* is essential for viral replication (transactivating factor) acting both on transcription and post-transcriptional modification of all viral proteins. *Art* acts to enhance the synthesis of viral structural proteins by promoting active translation of viral mRNA.
7. HIV chiefly infects cells bearing $CD_4$ receptors; gp 120 virus projections bind to $CD_4$ receptors on T-helper lymphocytes. The virus then enters the target cell by fusing directly with host cell membrane. (Fig. 3.1)
8. A double stranded DNA (provirus) is formed from viral RNA utilizing the enzyme reverse transcriptase. The provirus integrates into host cell's DNA and remains sequestered from host immune defences.
9. Mitogens, antigens, and cytokines such as tumour necrosis factor alpha, IL-6, and granulocyte-macrophage colony stimulating factor (GM-CSF) may induce the active replication of the latent virus, when new viruses bud out from the host cell membrane.
10. The newly formed gp 120 spikes bind to surrounding $CD_4$ molecules on adjacent cells, and hole their membrane. The punctured cells swell and die. Syncytium may form when the gp 120 of infected cell binds to $CD_4$ receptor or healthy cells. Thus many cells fuse to form the giant cell "Syncytium". Syncytia die soon after formation.

## NATURAL HISTORY OF HIV INFECTION

Usually, there is a period of 8 to 10 years from initial infection to clinical AIDS in adults, though AIDS may be manifested in less than two years or be delayed in onset beyond 10 years. It is clear that the longer an individual is infected, the more likely is the development of illness and subsequent death. Thus, HIV infection does not follow the pattern of more traditional viral diseases in which the risk of serious illness or death decreases with time. Primary HIV infection, also known as acute retroviral syndrome, may produce a mild and self-limited disease in 50 to 90% of persons infected with HIV. The time from exposure to development of symptoms averages 2 to 6 weeks. The symptoms may persist for 1 to 2 weeks, after which symptoms subside gradually. Prospective studies of acute HIV infections show that fever, fatigue, arthralgia or myalgia, lymphadenopathy, pharyngitis, diffuse erythematous macular or mixed maculopapular rash diarrhea, nausea or vomiting, weight loss, night sweats, mucocutaneous ulcerations, and headache are the most common symptoms seen with acute HIV infection.

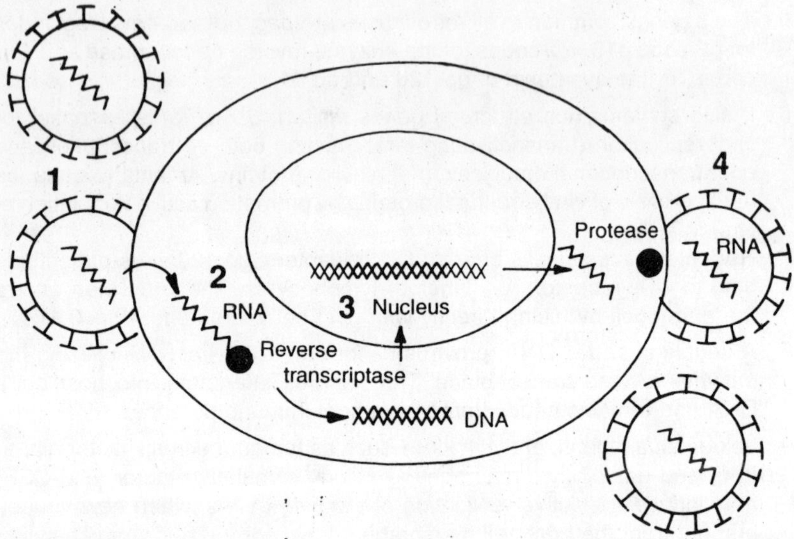


1. HIV enters a CD4 cell.
2. HIV is a retrovirus, To replicate, HIV uses an enzyme known as reverse transcriptase to convert its RNA into DNA.
3. HIV DNA enters the CD4 cell nucleus and inserts itself into the cell's DNA. HIV DNA then instructs the cell to make several copies of the original virus.
4. With the help of the protease enzyme, new virus particles are assembled. These newly formed viruses leave the cell, ready to infect other CD4 cells.

**Fig. 3.1. Stages of HIV reproduction** (CIPLA Teaching aid)

In the acute phase of HIV infection, (Fig. 3.2) there is active viral replication, particularly in CD4 lymphocytes, and a marked HIV viremia. This peripheral blood viremia is often in the range of 1,000,000 to 10,000,000 copies/mL of HIV-1 RNA. High titers of cytopathic HIV are detectable in the blood so that the p24 antigen test is usually positive, while HIV antibody tests (such as enzyme immunoassay) are often negative in the first three weeks. The viremia is greater in persons whose primary HIV infection is symptomatic. During this viremic phase, HIV disseminates throughout the body to lymphoid tissues and other organs such as brain. There are alterations in peripheral blood mononuclear cells marked by a decline in CD4+ lymphocytes. Persons acutely infected with HIV are highly infectious due to the high levels of HIV, both in blood as well as in genital secretions. Over half of all HIV infections may be transmitted during this period.

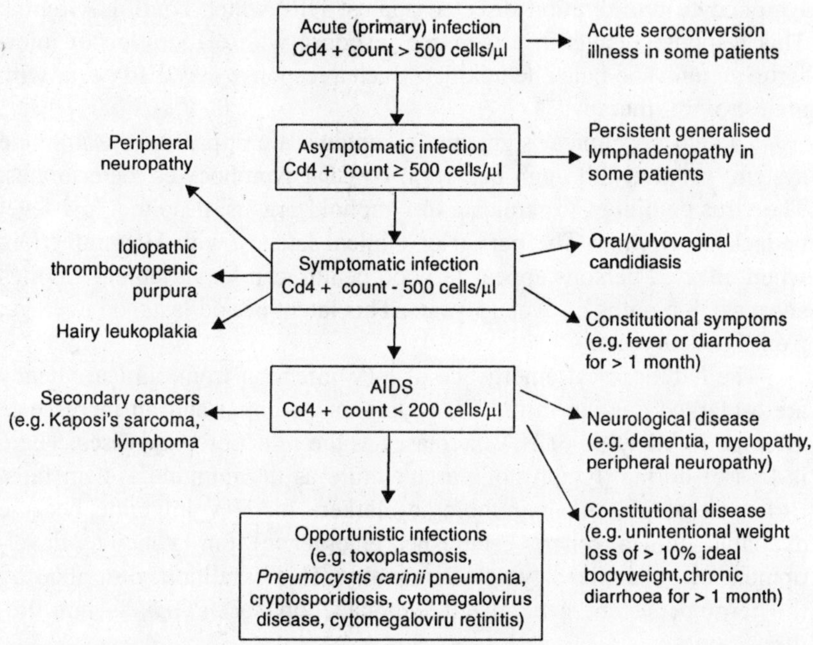


**Fig 3.2. Natural history of HIV infections.** (Current Medical Scene 2001; 16: 3)

Generally, within 3 weeks to 3 months following initial infection with HIV, the immune response is accompanied by a simultaneous decline in HIV viremia. Both humoral and cell mediated immune responses play a role. The CD4 lymphocytes rebound in number after primary HIV infection, but not to pre-infection levels. Seroconversion with detectable HIV antibody accompanies this immune response, sometimes in as little as a week, but more often in two to four weeks. The HIV infection then becomes clinically "latent". During this phase, there is little or no viral replication detectable in peripheral blood mononuclear cells and little or no culturable virus in peripheral blood. The CD4 lymphocyte count remains moderately decreased. However, the immune response to HIV is insufficient to prevent continued viral replication within lymphoid tissues. Tests for HIV antibody will remain positive during this time but p24 antigen tests are usually negative.

In other viral infections, an immune response consisting of virus-specific CD4 lymphocytes helps to contain the infection. However, such a response is typically lacking in HIV-infected persons. A minority of HIV-infected persons, however, do mount a persistent polyclonal CD4 lymphocyte proliferation directed against HIV which controls viremia. This response results in a cytokine response with elaboration of interferon gamma and beta chemokines. Such a response may also occur with antiretroviral therapy.

Though no clinical signs and symptoms are apparent, the immune system, primarily through depletion of CD4 lymphocytes, deteriorates. The virus continues to replicate in lymphoid organs, despite a low level or lack of viremia. The period of clinical latency with HIV infection, when infected persons appear in good health, can be variable – from as short as 18 months of over 15 years. This latent period lasts, on average, from 8 to 10 years.

The hallmarks of emergence of HIV infection from clinical latency are a marked decline in the CD4 lymphocyte count and an increase in viremia. Replication of HIV increases as the infection progresses. There is loss of normal lymph node architecture as the immune system fails. Before serologic and immunologic markers for HIV infection became available, clinical criteria established emergence from latency by development of generalized lymphadenopathy. This condition, described by the term persistent generalized lymphadenopathy (PGL), is not life-threatening.

Another phase of HIV infection described clinically but no longer commonly diagnosed in practice, is the condition known as AIDS-related complex (ARC), which is not necessarily preceded by PGL. ARC lacks only the opportunistic infections and neoplasms which define AIDS. ARC patients usually show symptoms of fatigue, weight loss, and night sweats, along with superficial fungal infections of the mouth and nails (See Chapter 9).

The ultimate stage of clinical AIDS reached years after initial infection is marked by the appearance of one or more of the typical opportunistic infections or neoplasms diagnostic of AIDS by definitional criteria. The progression to clinical AIDS is also marked by the appearance of syncytia-forming (SI) variants of HIV in about half of HIV infected patients. These SI viral variants, derived from non-syncytia-forming (NSI) variants, have greater CD4+ cell tropism and are associated with more rapid CD4+ cell decline.

**Table 3.3: Sub types of HIV-1**

| | | |
|---|---|---|
| Group M | | |
| • | Subtype A | Central Africa |
| • | Subtype B | South America (including Brazil), United States, Europe, Thailand |
| • | Subtype C | Brazil, India, Southern Africa |
| • | Subtype D | Central Africa |
| • | Subtype E | Thailand, Central African Republic |
| • | Subtype F | Brazil, Romania, Zaire |
| • | Subtype G | Zaire, Gabon, Thailand |
| • | Subtype H | Zaire, Gabon |
| Group N | | Cameroon |
| Group O | | West Africa |

Groups of HIV-1 and the subtype of group M of HIV are depicted in table 3.3 along with the geographic areas. HIV-I subtypes can undergo recombination to new strains which have different biological properties from original strains.

## Other human Retroviruses

**HIV-2:** A new retrovirus has been isolated from several patients with AIDS, initially from West African Countries and later on from Western Europe, the united States and elsewhere. It is designated as HIV-2. It spreads in a manner similar to HIV-1. Its high risk groups are commercial sex workers and sexually transmitted disease patients. Just as HIV-1 has distinct subtypes, so does HIV-2. The subtypes of HIV-2 have been designated from A through F. There is up to a 25% difference in genetic homology among these subtypes. All five subtypes can be detected by enzyme immunoassay (EIA) and Western blot assays for HIV-2 similar to those for HIV-1. Infection with HIV-2 eventually leads to AIDS. Persons can be coinfected with HIV-1 and HIV-2.

The natural history of HIV-2 infection is characterized by a longer latent period before the appearance of AIDS, a less aggressive course of AIDS, and a lower viral load with higher CD4 lymphocyte counts than HIV-1 infection until late in the course of the disease when clinical AIDS is apparent. Thus, the pathogenicity of HIV-2 appears to be lower than that of HIV-1. This may explain the more limited spread of HIV-2, compared to HIV-1, both in West African countries and elsewhere.

**Human T-cell leukemia virus (HTLV):** Another group of human retroviruses different from HIV are the human T-lymphotrophic viruses, types 1 and 2 (HTLV-1 and HTLV-2). Along with simian T-cell lymphoma virus type 1, they constitute a group of retroviruses known as the primate T-cell leukemia/lymphoma viruses. HTLV's can be transmitted in the same manner as HIV, though even less efficiently. Persons can be co-infected with HIV and HTLV. The CD4 lymphocytes are the cells primarily infected by HTLV. Laboratory testing methodology of HTLV's is similar to that for HIV. The enzyme immunoassay test for HTLV-1 will also detect HTLV-2. Confirmatory Western blot testing, in combination with testing for the presence of envelope peptide p21 helps to distinguish HTLV-1 from HTLV-2.

HTLV-1 infection is widespread in tropical and subtropical regions, with the main endemic foci in the Caribbean, southern Japan, central Africa, South Africa, and South America, particularly Brazil. Other endemic foci are found in southern India, northern Iran, aboriginal populations of northern Australia, and islands in the tropics. In Europe and North America, HTLV-1 infection is primarily associated with injection drug users and with immigrants from endemic areas. It is associated with adult T-cell leukemia/lymphoma (ATLL), with a form of chronic progressive neurologic disease known as HTLV-associated myelopathy/tropical spastic paraparesis (HAM/TSP), and with inflammatory conditions including polymyositis, arthropathy, infective dermatitis, and uveitis. The time from exposure to onset of HTLV-1 related disease is long – from 2 to 3 decades on average.

HTLV-2 is found as an endemic infection in the native peoples of the New World and pygmy tribes of Africa. In other populations, the spread of HTLV-2 occurs primarily as a result of injection drug use, particularly in metropolitan areas. There is no clear association between HTLV-2 and HTLL, but chronic neurologic disease, particularly spinocerebellar syndrome, may be linked to HTLV-2 infection.

# 4

# The Clinical Features

As evident from name, AIDS denotes an acquired immunodeficiency state of the body. The clinical reflection of this syndrome, thus, will only be secondary changes that will supervene in a gradually immuno-compromising host. So, it shares certain presentations of any congenital or acquired immunodeficiency, at the same time retain certain characteristic features of its own. The spectrum of AIDS (Fig. 4.1) can be visualised to be occupied at one end by the high-risk reservoir constituted by homosexual men, parentral drug abusers, haemophiliacs, Haitians, heterosexual partners of AIDS patients and their offsprings, having subclinical immunologic abnormalities, while the other end is formed by full-blown AIDS. The gap is bridged by persistent generalised lymphadenopathy, lesser AIDS and AIDS-related complex. Major manifestation of AIDS are bizarre malignancies and opportunistic infections. In addition, certain dermalogic presentations may also be observed. Of the odd neoplasms that develop in AIDS, Kaposi's sarcoma dominate the scene. The opportunistic infections observed in AIDS show certain peculiarities. Certain organisms affect AIDS patients more frequently than other immunocompromised hosts. Every infection presents a more or less distinct clinical picture. However, more often than not, an extensive multi-systematic involvement may be caused by an invading pathogen, thus producing widespread, non-localising signs and symptoms. The confusion may further be compounded if many organisms have attacked such a host. In this case, the etiology of a group of symptoms may be multiple with the result that the patient does not respond, if the therapy is directed against a single microbe. These infections have been dealt with separately in details in Chapter 7. They cause alarming rise in mortality in AIDS patients.

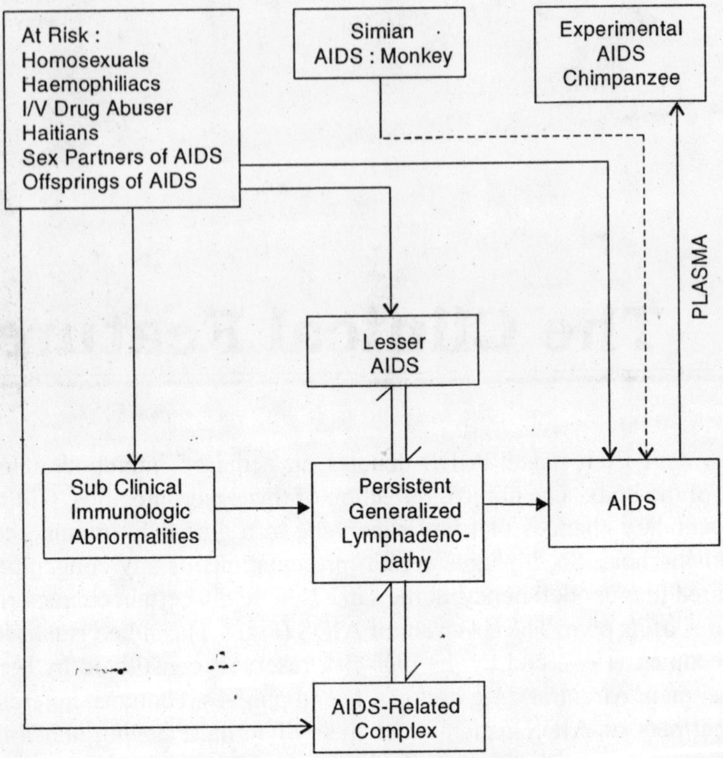


**Fig. 4.1. The Spectrum of AIDS**

The Centres for Disease Control classification of HIV-infection (1986) has divided it into 4 groups (Table 4.1).

**Table 4.1: Centres for Disease Control classification of HIV disease**

| | |
|---|---|
| Group I | Acute infection |
| Group II | Asymptomatic infection |
| Group III | Persistent generalised lymphadenopathy |
| Group IV | |
| A: | Constitutional disease (as in AIDS-related complex) |
| B: | Neuological disease (HIV encephalopathy defines AIDS) |
| C: | Secondary infectious disease |
| | 1 – Those defining AIDS |
| | 2 – Others |
| D: | Malignancy secondary to HIV disease (thus defining AIDS) |
| E: | Other conditions |

**I** The acute infection, usually asymptomatic, but in upto 50% of people can cause a glandular fever-like illness (discussed under natural history). At this stage p24 antigen is detectable in the blood, usually for a week or two, but antibodies have yet to appear. An antibody response to both p24 and gp41 antigens follows.

**II** A prolonged asymptomatic period which can last for many years during which antibodies to both p24 and gp41 persist (range from 2 months to 7 years or longer; mean 2½ years). Early signs of neurological dysfunction may be detected towards the end of this stage.

**III** Persistent generalised lymphadenopathy mark this phase, but there are no other signs or symptoms of infection. This is defined as lymph node enlargement in two or more extra-inguinal sites for at least 3 months. The nodes are typically rubbery, mobile and intermittently tender. Antibodies to both p24 and gp41 are detectable.

**IV** Symptomatic disease: At the beginning of this phase, there may be a decline and disappearance of p24 antigen in the blood; antibody to gp41 continues to be produced. It is subdivided according to the clinical manifestations into subgroups A to E. The majority of group IV patients have decreased numbers of T-helper cells, usually below 100/mm$^3$.

Progressive impairment of immune function will lead the full-blown AIDS, defined as occurrence of a major disease indicative of a defect in cell-mediated immunity in a patient with no known cause for immunodeficiency other than HIV infection. The great majority of such patients are seropositive for HIV. Seropositivity however, is not essential for the diagnosis. Relevant diseases include protozoal, fungal, viral, mycobacterial (and less commonly other bacterial) infections; certain malignancies especially Kaposi's sarcoma and non-Hodgkin lymphomas; and HIV infection of the central nervous system. Estimates of the average time between acquisition of HIV and the onset of AIDS are around 8 to 11 years. The proportion of HIV-infected patients who eventually develop AIDS is not yet known, but of the homosexual men in the San Franciscan study, 54% had AIDS within 10 years of seroconversion, and about half of the recipients of HIV-contaminated blood developed AIDS within 7 years. Patients with AIDS usually die from opportunistic infection, CNS disease or wasting; less commonly from malignancy. A thorough physical examination is mandatory in all cases (Table 4.2).

## CUTANEOUS MARKERS

The dermatologic manifestations of AIDS patients, apart from Kaposi's sarcoma, include the following entities:

**Seborrhoeic dermatitis:** The seborrhoeic-like dermatitis of AIDS bears certain distinctions from the usual form. It is more explosive and shows more angry looking lesions, characterised by thick, greasy, hyperkeratotic plaques with underlying inflammation. Sites of involvement are however seborrhoeic sites (scalp, face, chest) of the body. The histopathology of AIDS-related seborrhoeic dermatitis is equally characteristic, and is comprised of widespread parakeratosis, scattered necrotic keratinocytes, thick-walled blood vessels in the dermis, numerous plasma cells and focal leukocytoclasia. This appears to be a distinct clinical entity of unknown origin, mimicking seborrhoeic dermatitis.

**Table 4.2: Physical examination baseline evaluation**

The goal is screening for active problems, clues to disease stage and documenting baseline values.

*Vital signs:* Baseline vital signs (weight, blood pressure, pulse rate, temperature, respiratory rate)

*Eyes:* Baseline extraocular movement, pupil size, reactivity, retinal examination.

*Oropharynx:* missing, tender or decaying teeth; gum inflammation or tenderness; appearance of pharyngeal lymphoid tissue; oral candidiasis; hairy leukoplakia; pigmented lesions; exudates.

*Pulmonary Cardiac:* As for any primary care examination.

*Abdominal:* Organomegaly, masses, focal tenderness.

*Genitalia:* Condylomata, ulcers, abnormalities beneath foreskin, discharge, testicular lesions or atrophy.

*Pelvic:* Vaginal discharge, inflammation, cervical lesions, masses, tenderness, Pap smear for dysplasia, STD cultures if appropriate.

*Rectal:* Condylomata, ulcers, mass lesions, tenderness.

*Skin:* Fungal infections (periungual, feet, groin, axilla), oedema, nodules, condylomata, pigmented lesions (Kaposi's sarcoma).

*Lymph nodes:* Enlargement (document size), asymmetric or focal enlargement, tenderness.

*Neurologic:* Careful baseline examination.

*Mental status:* Consider evaluation of mental status.

In most cases topical imidazoles alone or with a topical steroid will control the eruption. Thick scalp scales may require overnight treatment with sulphur-salicyclic acid creams or 1.5% salicyclic acid in arachis oil. In difficult cases an oral imidazole may be justified especially if there is co-existing candidiasis.

**Butterfly eruptions.** They can commonly be seen in AIDS patients, simulating the rash of lupus erythematosus. Papular eruptions may also be observed over head, neck and upper trunk. They are mildly pruritic. Extensive lesions may present as acneiform folliculitis. Microscopic examination reveals granuloma formation in perivascular/perifollicular pattern. These eruptions may result from an aberrant immunologic reaction to skin saprophytes or dermatophytes, as sometimes *Demodex folliculorum* or dermatophytes can be demonstrated.

**Bacillary (epithelioid) angiomatosis.** Angioma-like lesions affecting skin, mucosal surfaces and internal organs, typically begin as tiny pinpoint papules, often widespread and in large numbers. They may enlarge to papules and nodules, resembling AIDS -related Kaposi's sarcoma (the two may coexist), but the macules and plaques seen in the latter do not occur. If injured, lesions bleed profusely. Visceral lesions may occur, and deaths from laryngeal obstruction and disseminated intravascular obstruction are not uncommon. It is seen mainly in HIV disease, but may also occur in other immunodeficient patients. The condition responds well to erythromycin (1-2 g daily), given for several weeks. It is caused by an argyrophilic bacillus, similar to the cat scratch disease bacillus, but the two bacteria are not identical.

**Yellow nail syndrome.** A yellow discolouration of distal parts of nail has been observed in some AIDS patients, associated with longitudinal and transverse ridging. Onycholysis may occur. These patients usually show chest afflictions, especially *P. carinii* pneumonia. Classic yellow nail syndrome, on the other hand, is usually associated with chronic respiratory infections with lymphoedema.

**Xeroderma simulating ichthyosiform dermatitis.** This is usually a feature of chronic, wasting illnesses including malignancies and malabsorption syndrome. Its occurrence in AIDS may reflect similar nutritional deficiencies. Paediatric AIDS usually show this change.

**Papulopruritic eruption (itchy folliculitis).** Small, often extremely itchy red or skin-coloured papules on the head, neck and trunk are common in HIV disease, distinct from recognised causes of folliculitis (including pyogenic bacterial infection, acneiform eruptions, pityrosporum folliculitis and demodicidosis). The histology shows a rather non-specific, mainly perifollicular, mixed cell infiltrate, but some cases of what appear to be the same condition also show granuloma formation or a vasculitis with follicular necrosis. The cause is not clear, but a sensitization reaction to an infection at some distant site has been suggested.

Treatment with antimicrobials, antihistamines, and topical steroids has little effect, but UVB and PUVA have helped some patients, though relapse is common if treatment is stopped.

**Hyperalgesic pseudothrombophlebitis syndrome.** It has been observed in some homosexual men with Kaposi's sarcoma. It presents with a painful swelling of the calf with positive Homan's sign. It mimics deep vein thrombosis as the overlying skin becomes erythematous, oedematous and exquisitely tender. No evidence of venous occlusion can, however, be seen on venography. Gradual spontaneous resolution starts in 1-4 weeks, and completes in several weeks.

**Oral hairy leukoplakia.** It is primarily seen on the lateral borders of the tongue, as mildly raised, poorly demarcated plaques with corrugated (hairy) surface. Histopathological examination demonstrates a picture similar to that observed in warty or condylomatous lesions. This condition may sometimes precede AIDS by several weeks or months.

Candidiasis may coexist but is not the cause. Treatment is not always indicated unless there is significant discomfort. Systemic acyclovir (400 mg five times daily orally), ganciclovir and foscarnet and topical acyclovir and tretinoin have led to its regression. Surgical excision of individual lesions is feasible.

**Prurigo-like lesions.** These lesions, distinct from papulopruritic eruption, were recorded in 46% of 134 Haitian HIV patients, and have been described in Central Africa as well. The lesions cleared when patients went to the USA and recurred on their return to deficiency. It began on the extensor surfaces of the arms and became widespread, and was intensely itchy. No useful treatment was found.

**Gingivitis.** This is common in HIV disease. More severe bacterial involvement may lead to ulceration and even to *gangrenous stomatitis,* a severe mixed bacterial infection of oral tissues occurring in immunosuppressed or debilitated patients. Treatment includes antibiotics (e.g. penicillin and metronidazole), intraoral antiseptics, vigorous dental hygiene and occasionally removal of teeth and necrotic bone.

**Cytomegalovirus (CMV).** A common cause of retinal, gastro-intestinal and lung infection in AIDS, CMV may occasionally give rise to one or more persistent keratotic skin lesions. Viral inclusions may be seen histologically and virus may be cultured from biopsy tissue. Other eruptions attributed to CMV include vasculitis, perianal and oral ulceration, indurated pigmented nodules and plaques and vesiculobullous lesions.

**Immune complex vasculitis.** An immune complex vasculitis associated with purpura can be seen in some AIDS patients. This histopathologically suggests a leukocytoclastic pattern, while special procedures reveal the presence of immunofluoroscence when serum with high titres of HIV-1 are used, suggesting that this virus is the source of antigen in this immune complex phenomenon.

**Cutaneous anergy to standard test antigens.** Delayed hypersensitivity, which is intact early in the syndrome, gradually wanes off, reflecting as cutaneous anergy to various standard test antigens, primarily due to suppression of cellular immunity.

**Other skin manifestations.** A variety of viral, fungal and bacterial infections can develop over the skin of infection-prone AIDS victims. Norwegian scabies is also occasionally reported. Of the cutaneous viral infections, herpes simplex, herpes zoster, molluscum contagiosum, warts and condyloma acuminata are notably seen in AIDS. They are unusually extensive and may frequently recur after treatment. The fungal infections commonly affecting skin and mucous membranes of AIDS patients are candidiasis, and sometimes cryptococcosis. Apart from the involvement of integument, they may also cause widespread systemic damage. Pyogenic bacteria also get their dues, causing streptococcal/staphylococcal pyo-dermas, folliculitis, and so on. Malignant syphilis can prove fatal.

**Fat Redistribution Syndrome.** A consistent syndrome of body fat redistribution is seen in HIV-positive patients. A characteristic pattern of fat loss in the cheeks is very common. Other abnormalities of the adipose tissue include benign symmetric lepomatosis, breast hypertrophy, thinning of thighs and buttocks, accumulation of visceral abdominal fat, buffalo hump, lipodystrophy and cushingoid features.

## PSYCHOSOCIAL ISSUE

The tremendous stigma and terror associated with the word AIDS obviously cause a major handicap in the hitherto smooth sailing social life of these patients, once they are labelled as AIDS. It can be compared with the phobias and stigmas once used to be attached to the word leper. Leprosy, unlike AIDS, is not a rapidly fatal disease. AIDS, on the other hand, shatters all hopes of the afflicted subject, as the patients themselves know that there is as yet no cure for AIDS. Numerous instances have occurred where homosexuals or drug abusers committed suicide, suspecting them to be suffering from AIDS. Naturally one can not conceive, and thus acclimatize the transformation from a young, agile healthy person to a debilitated, nearly dying man, full of nerve-wrecking symptoms, in just a matter of months.

The first responsibility of the treating physician emerges at the time of diagnosis of the disease. This is the most crucial period, and a label of AIDS can adversely affect the patients' as well as their relations' life. Thus, it goes without saying that the caption AIDS should only be given to those patients who have unequivocal clinical and laboratory pointers towards AIDS. The laboratory, in particular, should be manned by staff who are experienced enough in meticulously carrying out these procedures.

The patient undergoes a complex chain of stresses and strains, both physical and psychological, from the onset of AIDS till its fulminant end. Further, they usually respond adversely to the therapy as well. After they know that they are suffering from an intractable illness that will disfigure their body, give extreme agony, and ultimately kill them mercilessly, they have to live every second of this nightmare in reality, waiting with panic what will happen the next day. They are obsessed with a feeling of utter insecurity and loneliness. These phobias of disfigurement, debili-tation, infections, cancers and pangs of death are compounded by the fear of social abandonment, humiliation and guilt about their past sexual behaviours. Additional problems are created by the loss of their sexual relationship on which they used to have built their centres of interpersonal relationship. Loss of employment may be equally distressing.

Profound psychiatric complications of AIDS have been a regular feature in most established cases. The psychiatric aspects of AIDS can, thus, be classified into two broad areas:

(i) The various ways in which AIDS manifests as psychiatric syndromes, and
(ii) The impact on the individual, his family, society and professionals involved in his care.

A variety of neuropsychiatric and functional disorders have been described which affect HIV-infected individuals at various stages. Dementia, delirium, organic mental disorders, affective illness, delusional and schizophreniform psychosis, anxiety, adjustment problems and various emotional reactions are not uncommon.

The general principles of counselling and psychotherapy should be used in the management of psychological problems among patients with AIDS. Providing a good human relationship from the basis of therapy. Information and education for these individuals on the nature of the illness, its prognosis and treatment, its prevention and other related issues are important. Instruction on safer sexual practices and counselling for drug abusers are important in its prevention. Psychological intervention for emotional problems arising as reaction to the illness would be crucial in its overall management. Individual and group therapy for patients and their families have been providing psychological help to the affected individuals. Supportive and cognitive therapies are useful in tackling the problems faced by these individuals. Psychodynamic and behavioural approaches are also recommended.

# 5

# Pediatric – HIV Infection/AIDS

Pediatric HIV infection/AIDS has important clinical differences, which, taken with the lack of simple laboratory tests in infancy, make the diagnosis less easy to confirm, although AIDS in children has many similarities to that in adult. The presence of HIV antibody (IgG) in infancy may simply represent passively acquired maternal antibody, and cannot be used as an indication of HIV infection. In one study, of 117 children of HIV-seropositive mothers tested at 18 months, 65% were seronegative and well, and 27% had serological evidence of HIV infection; however the remaining 8% were seronegative but had clinical or laboratory features suggesting HIV infection, so that loss of antibody does not always indicate absence of HIV infection. Circulating HIV antigen is likely to be obscured by maternal antibody. Pediatric HIV infection is primarily acquired perinatally. The infection can occur *in utero* prior to birth, intrapartum during delivery or via breast milk following delivery. Worldwide approximately 1800 HIV infected infants are born each day. Other causes of pediatric HIV infection uncommonly seen are sexual abuse or blood transfusion. The later is rare now a days because of adequate testing of blood. In India, there were 749 pediatric AIDS cases amongst 20,304 total AIDS patients from May 1986 till March 2001 (NACO, 2002). There were 470 boys and 279 girls.

## CLINICAL FEATURES

Around 14 to 25% of children are born to HIV-1 infected mothers are perinatally infected in the United States and Europe, while the figure is about 13 to 42% in the developing nations. However, the rate of HIV infection in the firstborn of twins delivered vaginally (35%) is greater than the rate in second born (15%). Further, 15% rate of HIV infection in the firstborn of twins delivered by cesarean section is greater than the 8% rate for the second born, suggesting that intrapartum HIV infection does occur. A greater HIV viral burden in the mother during late gestation and/or during the time of delivery, as measured by HIV-1 RNA levels, increases the risk for HIV transmission to the baby. The risk is increased with preterm labor and premature rupture of membranes. The risk is halved with delivery by elective cesarean section. For mothers with HIV-2 infection, the rate of perinatal transmission is only 1 to 2 per cent. Breast feeding by HIV-infected mothers further increases the risk for transmission of HIV to an infant.

Zidovudine therapy in an HIV-infected mother has been shown to reduce the rate of perinatal transmission of HIV by two-thirds. Zidovudine decreases viral load and decreases the risk for perinatal transmission in late gestation and/or at the time of delivery. Such therapy includes antenatal maternal oral administration of zidovudine starting at 14 to 34 weeks gestation and continuing throughout the pregnancy, intravenous maternal zidovudine therapy during labor and delivery, and oral administration of zidovudine to the infant 8 to 12 hours after birth and continuing for 6 weeks following delivery. No association with birth defects has been reported from zidovudine therapy.

Two patterns of progression to AIDS with perinatal HIV infection are usually seen. In about 10 to 25% infections, the infants and children manifest severe immunodeficiency with failure to thrive and encephalopathy in the first two years of life, with nearly 100% mortality from AIDS by 4 years of age. Rapid progression of perinatally acquired HIV-1 may be predicted by a number of factors. These include positive HIV-1 culture or polymerase chain reaction (PCR) assay during the first week of life, < 30% CD4+T-lymphocytes at birth, and any or all of the following noted at birth: hepatomegaly, splenomegaly and lymphadenopathy. Specific infectious diseases, severe bacterial infections, progressive neurologic disease, anemia, fever, cardiomyopathy, growth failure, hepatitis, and persistent oral candidiasis contribute to shortened survival. In the remaining 75 to 90% cases, children with HIV infection have a much slower progression to AIDS over 10 years or more, often remaining asymptomatic through adolescence, and their morbidity and mortality more closely resembles that of adult AIDS.

In the developed nations, most of the mothers of infants with HIV infection have acquired HIV infection as intravenous drug users or as sexual partners of drug users, but increasing numbers of mothers are currently acquiring HIV heterosexually. In addition, some sexually abused children have contracted AIDS, with symptoms often not appearing until adolescence. Transfusion-associated AIDS in the early 1980's accounted for about 10% of pediatric cases and transfusion of blood products for hemophilia about 5%. In places where screening of blood products for HIV has been employed, these percentages have decreased substantially. Death has occurred in over 75% of reported pediatric AIDS cases, usually with opportunistic infections similar to adult AIDS patients, but with a clinical course, on overall average, shorter than that of adult patients. The prominent clinical features in pediatric HIV infection are enumerated below.

## Failure to Thrive

Poor growth may be seen in up to half of HIV-infected children. The decrease in growth continues over time, and appears to involve lean body mass. This effect may be present from birth, since it is noted that infants born to HIV-infected mothers (even those who do not acquire HIV) have a significantly lower mean birth weight and length. Micronutrient deficiencies, and vitamin A deficiency, may play a role, but dietary supplementation does not correct deficits in lean body mass or height. The levels of HIV-1 RNA are higher in children with poor growth.

## Pulmonary Features

Pulmonary problems include *Pneumocystis carinii* (PCP), which occurs in over half of pediatric patients with AIDS, and has a high mortality rate in infants less than 2 months of age. Around 12% of infants with perinatally acquired HIV infection develop PCP in the first year of life. More than a third of pediatric AIDS patients die from PCP. Recurrent bacterial infections are common and account for about 20% of deaths from AIDS in children. Prophylaxis is recommended for all infants with perinatal HIV exposure, beginning at 4 to 6 weeks of life, and continuing throughout the first year of life if HIV infection is confirmed. Despite prophylaxis, PCP may still occur. The risk of PCP is increased when the CD4 count is declining or when maternal CD4 counts are lower, but does not appear to be related to HIV-1 RNA levels.

Lymphoid interstitial pneumonitis (LIP) is not characteristic of adult AIDS but is seen occasionally in about 20% of all children with AIDS. LIP rarely causes death and affected children may have a better prognosis than that of HIV-infected children with other opportunistic infections and neoplasms. It usually develops when passively acquired maternal antibody begins to disappear. Cytomegalovirus infection of the lungs is also common and may be associated with pulmonary failure and death. Mycobacterial and fungal infections are uncommon.

A polyclonal B-cell lymphoproliferative disorder (PBLD) can also affect the lungs in children with HIV infection, along with other sites including liver, spleen, lymph nodes, and kidneys resulting in the patosplenomegaly and lymphadenopathy.

## CNS Features

The commonest neurological finding in pediatric HIV infection is progressive encephalopathy due to invasion of HIV-1 in the central nervous system. It affects 30 to 60 percent of pediatric AIDS patients. Human immunodeficiency virus-associated dementia (HIVD)/AIDS-dementia complex shows 3 major patterns depicted in the table 5.1.

**Table 5.1: Major patterns of AIDS-dementia complex**

| Pattern | Feature(s) |
|---|---|
| 1. Subacute Progressive | Initial normal development; subsequently, social language and motor skills are lost. Microcephaly is seen. |
| 2. Plateau Progressive | Initial Development at normal pace, followed by decline in their rate of developmental progress with little or no further acquisition of skill. Microcephaly is seen. |
| 3. Static encephalopathy | Motor and language skills are acquired slowly, children are cognitively impaired; Acquire skills slowly. Scans are normal. |

Other features are acquired microcephaly with decreased brain weight accompanied with ventriculomegaly and cortical atrophy. Children with encephalopathy often have corticospinal tract degeneration from myelin loss. Vacuolar myelopathy as seen in spinal cords of adults is uncommon. An anoxic-ischemic encephalopathy with neuronal necrosis in cerebral cortex, hippocampus, and basal ganglia may be seen in association with systemic hypoxemia from cardiovascular disease. Although non-Hodgkin's lymphoma can be seen in pediatric AIDS patients with focal CNS lesions, opportunistic infections such as toxoplasmosis, cryptococcosis, cytomegalovirus, and progressive multifocal leukoencephalopathy are uncommon in pediatric AIDS, in contrast to the adult AIDS.

## Neoplasia

Pediatric AIDS has less incidence of neoplasms compared to AIDS. The incidence of malignant neoplasms are around 2.5 per cent. A high grade non-Hodkins lymphoma (NHL) is the most frequent neoplasm seen in HIV infected children. Clinical findings seen at presentation with NHL's in pediatric AIDS include fever, weight loss, jaundice, hepato-splenomegaly, abdominal distension, anemia, and neurologic abnormalities. Most patients are at stage III or IV on presentation. NHL's are more likely to occur in boys who are Caucasians and who are older. Brain lymphomas tend to occur late in the course of AIDS. Mucosa-associated lymphoid tissue (MALT) lesions have been seen in association with pediatric HIV infection. They are characteristically localized and found in lung, salivary gland, and tonsils.

The Kaposi's sarcoma is less frequent than seen in adult AIDS and is seen at the age between 5 and 6 years. Next in frequency are smooth muscle tumors, leiomyomas or leiomyosarcomas, the latter being the second leading cancer in children with HIV infection. These tumors are generally visceral in location (gastrointestinal tract, lung, spleen, and liver). In lung, the lesions appear as multiple nodules; tracheobroncial involvement may lead to respiratory distress with wheezing. Gastrointestinal lesions may produce bloody diarrhea, abdominal pain, and obstruction. Epstein-Barr virus can be demonstrated in the cells of HIV-associated smooth muscle neoplasms, and EBV stimulated clonal proliferation may contribute to their pathogenesis in both children as well as adults.

## Other important features

Human immunodeficiency virus nephropathy (HIVN) can occur in children with HIV infection, with excessive proteinuria or albuminuria. Focal and segmental glomerulosclerosis (FSGS) is seen in only half of cases, and other changes may include mesangial hyperplasia. The course in children is less fulminant than in adults, still they may progress to end-stage renal disease.

The thymus in pediatric AIDS undergoes marked involution with apparent irreversible injury that contributes to immunosuppression. Thymic depletion may result in immune dysfunction and subsequently more rapid progression of disease with HIV infection. Findings in the thymus at autopsy in pediatric patients with HIV infection, who died from AIDS, may include severe lymphoid depletion with atrophy, microcystic transformation and/or calcification of Hassall's corpuscles, plasma cell infiltrates, and Warthin-Finkeldey type giant cells.

An arteriopathy has been described at autopsy in children dying of AIDS in which there is either cerebral vasculitis or generalized fibrocalcific change in elastic lamina or media of arteries in brain, lung, thymus, kidney, spleen, heart, and lymph node. The lumenal narrowing may explain focal necrosis, atrophy, fibrosis, or gliosis. In the brain, this arteriopathy is manifested as a diffuse dilation with ectasia of major arteries of the circle of Willis, with intimal fibroplasia, medial thinning, and elastic lamina destruction or reduplication. It can lead to hemorrhages in cerebrum, basal ganglia, and subarachnoid space. Infarctions may also occur. Though little inflammation is identified within these lesions at autopsy, the features suggest a prior vasculitis, and often a history of a prior opportunistic infection, particularly varicella zoster virus (VZV).

### Other infections

*Candida* infection of the esophagus or lung has been seen in 10% of pediatric cases. Recurrent oral thrush, a frequent finding in infants with AIDS, may give rise to invasive or systemic candidiasis. Systemic, recurrent bacterial infections are seen with increased frequency. Diarrhea can be a serious problem in HIV-infected infants. It has an earlier onset than in healthy infants, and tends to be more persistent. Fever, vomiting, anorexia, and dehydration often accompany the diarrheal illness. Often, pathogen cannot be found. The most common pathogens identified are cytomegalovirus, rotavirus and *salmonella* species.

Granulomas are seen less frequently in HIV-infected children and few organisms are present with either mycobacterial or fungal infections than in adult AIDS patients. The large histiocytes containing *Mycobacterium avium-intracellulare* found throughout the reticuloendothelial system in some cases may mimic the cells observed with some storage diseases such as Gaucher's disease and Niemann-Pick disease.

## DIAGNOSIS

The diagnosis of HIV infection in pediatric age-group especially newborn born to HIV infected mother is complicated by the presence of maternal anti-HIV-IgG antibodies which are able to cross Placenta. All these newborn are HIV-positive at birth, although only 15-30 per cent are actually infected. By the age of 9 months or occasionally upto 18 months, this antibody becomes undetectable in uninfected children. Polymerase chain reaction (PCR) and virus culture are probably the most sensitive and specific assays for detecting HIV-infection in children born to infected mothers, which are 30 to 50 percent specific at birth and nearly 100 per

**Table 5.2: Diagnosis of human immunodeficiency virus (HIV) infection in children* (MMWR 1994: 43: 1-10)**

**Diagnosis: HIV Infected**

(a) A child <18 months of age who is known to be HIV seropositive or born to an HIV-infected mother and:

- has positive results on two separate determinations (excluding cord blood) from one or more of the following HIV detection tests:
  - HIV culture,
  - HIV polymerase chain reaction,
  - HIV antigen (p24), or
- meets criteria for acquired immunodeficiency syndrome (AIDS) diagnosis based on the 1987 AIDS surveillance case definition.

(b) A child ≥ 18 months of age born to an HIV-infected mother or any child infected by blood, blood products, or other known modes of transmission (e.g., sexual contact) who:

- is HIV-antibody positive by repeatedly reactive enzyme immunoassay (EIA) and confirmatory test (e.g., Western blot or immunofluorescence assay [IFA]); or
- meets any of the criteria in a ) above.

**Diagnosis: Perinatally Exposed (Prefix E)**

A child who does not meet the criteria above who:

- is HIV seropositive by EIA and confirmatory test (e.g., Western blot or IFA) and is < 18 months of age at the time of test; or
- has unknown antibody status, but was born to a mother known to be infected with HIV.

**Diagnosis: Seroreverter (SR)**

A child who is born to an HIV-infected mother and who:

- has been documented as HIV-antibody negative (i.e., two or more negative EIA tests performed at 6-18 months of age or one negative EIA test after 18 months of age); and
- has had no other laboratory evidence of infection (has not had two positive viral detection tests, if performed); and
- has not had an AIDS-defining condition.

cent specific at 3-6 months of age (Table 5.2). Children born to mothers with HIV infection are defined as seroreverters (SRs) and are considered uninfected with HIV if they (a) become HIV-antibody negative after 6 months of age, (b) have no other laboratory evidence of HIV infection, and (c) have not met the AIDS surveillance case definition criteria.

Three immunologic categories have been established to categorise children according to severity of immunosuppression attributable to HIV (Table 5.3).

**Table 5.3: Immunologic categories based on age specific CD4 + T-cell count and percentage of total lymphocytes (MMWR 1994; 43: 1-10)**

| | Age of Child | | |
|---|---|---|---|
| Immunologic Category | < 1 year<br>µL (%) | 1-5 year<br>µL (%) | 6-12 year<br>µL (%) |
| 1. No evidence of Immuno-suppresion | ≥ 1500<br>(≥25) | ≥1000<br>(≥25) | ≥ 500<br>(≥25) |
| 2. Moderate immuno-suppression | 750-1499<br>(15-24) | 500-999<br>(15-24) | 200-499<br>(15-24) |
| 3. Severe immuno-suppression | 750<br>(< 15) | < 500<br>(< 15) | < 200<br>(< 15) |

Clinical Categories of HIV infected children are tabulated in Table 5.4.

**Table 5.4. Clinical categories for children with human immuno-deficiency virus (HIV) infection (MMWR 1994; 43:6)**

**Category N: Not Symptomatic**

Children who have no signs or symptoms considered to be the result of HIV infection or who have only one of the conditions listed in Category A.

**Category A: Mildly Symptomatic**

Children with two or more of the conditions listed below but none of the conditions listed in Categories B and C.

- Lymphadenopathy (≥ 0.5 cm at over two sites; bilateral = one site)
- Hepatomegaly
- Splenomegaly
- Dermatitis
- Parotitis

*(Contd.)*

*Table 5.4 (Contd.)*

- Recurrent or persistent upper respiratory infection, sinusitis, or otitis media

**Category B: Moderately symptomatic**

Children who have symptomatic conditions other than those listed for Category A or C that are attributed to HIV infection. Examples of conditions in clinical Category B include but are not limited to:

- Anemia (< 8 gm/dL), neutropenia (< 1,000/mm$^3$), or thrombocytopenia (< 100,000/mm$^3$) persisting ≥ 30 days
- Bacterial meningitis, pneumonia, or sepsis (single episode)
- Candidiasis, oropharyngeal (thrush), persisting (> 2 months) in children > 6 months of age
- Cardiomyopathy
- Cytomegalovirus infection, with onset before 1 month of age
- Diarrhea, recurrent or chronic
- Hepatitis
- Herpes simplex virus (HSV) stomatitis, recurrent (more than two episodes within 1 year)
- HSV bronchitis, pneumonitis, or esophagitis with onset before 1 month of age
- Herpes zoster (shingles) involving at least two distinct episodes or more than one dermatome
- Leiomyosarcoma
- Lymphoid interstitial pneumonia (LIP) or pulmonary lymphoid hyperplasia complex
- Nephropathy
- Nocardiosis
- Persistent fever (lasting > 1 month)
- Toxoplasmosis, onset before 1 month of age
- Varicella, disseminated (complicated chickenpox)

**Category C: Severely Symptomatic**

Children who have any condition listed in the 1987 surveillance case definition for acquired immunodeficiency syndrome, with the exception of LIP, eg.

- Serious bacterial infections, multiple or recurrent (i.e., any combination of at least two culture-confirmed infections within a 2-year period), of the following types: septicemia, pneumonia, meningitis, bone or joint infection, or abscess of an internal organ or body cavity (excluding otitis media, superficial skin or mucosal abscesses, and indwelling catheter-related infections)

*(Contd.)*

*Table 5.4 (Contd.)*

- Candidiasis, esophageal or pulmonary (bronchi, trachea, lungs)
- Coccidioidomycosis, disseminated (at site other than or in addition to lungs or cervical or hilar lymph nodes)
- Cryptococcosis, extrapulmonary
- Cryptosporidiosis or isosporiasis with diarrhea persisting > 1 month
- Cytomegalovirus disease with onset of symptoms at age > 1 month (at a site other than liver, spleen, or lymph nodes)
- Encephalopathy (at least one of the following progressive findings present for at least 2 months in the absence of a concurrent illness other than HIV infection that could explain the findings): a) failure to attain or loss of developmental milestones or loss of intellectual ability, verified by standard developmental scale or neuropsychological tests; b) impaired brain growth or acquired microcephaly demonstrated by head circumference measurements or brain atrophy demonstrated by computerized tomography or magnetic resonance imaging (serial imaging is required for children < 2 years of age); c) acquired symmetric motor deficit manifested by two or more of the following: paresis, pathologic reflexes, ataxia, or gait disturbance
- Herpes simplex virus infection causing a mucocutaneous ulcer that persists for > 1 month; or bronchitis, pneumonitis, or esophagitis for any duration affecting a child > 1 month of age
- Histoplasmosis, disseminated (at a site other than or in addition to lungs or cervical or hilar lymph nodes)
- Kaposi's sarcoma
- Lymphoma, primary, in brain
- Lymphoma, small, noncleaved cell (Burkitt's), or immunoblastic or large cell lymphoma of B-cell or unknown immunologic phenotype
- *Mycobacterium tuberculosis,* disseminated or extrapulmonary
- *Mycobacterium,* other species disseminated (at a site other than or in addition to lungs, skin, or cervical or hilar lymph nodes)
- *Mycobacterium avium* complex or *Mycobacterium kansasii,* disseminated (at site other than or in addition to lungs, skin, or cervical or hilar lymph nodes)
- *Pneumocystis carinii* pneumonia
- Progressive multifocal leukoencephalopathy
- Salmonella (nontyphoid) septicemia, recurrent
- Toxoplasmosis of the brain with onset at > 1 month of age
- Wasting syndrome in the absence of a concurrent illness other than HIV infection that could explain the following findings: a) persistent

*(Contd.)*

*Table 5.4 (Contd.)*

weight loss > 10% of baseline OR b) downward crossing of at least two of the following percentile lines on the weight-for-age chart (e.g., 95th, 75th, 50th, 25th, 5th) in a child ≥1 year of age OR c) <5th percentile on weight-for-height chart on two consecutive measurements, ≥30 days apart PLUS a) chronic diarrhea (i.e., at least two loose stools per day for ≥30 days) OR b) documented fever (for ≥30 days, intermittent or constant)

The subdivision of clinical categories virus immunologic categories further clarifies the picture of pediatric AIDS (Table 5.5)

**Table 5.5: Pediatric human immunodeficiency virus (HIV) classification* (MMWR 1994; 43:1-10)**

| | Clinical categories | | | |
|---|---|---|---|---|
| Immunologic categories | N: No signs/ symptoms | A: Mild signs/ symptoms | B: Moderate signs/ symptoms | C: Severe signs/ symptoms |
| 1. No evidence of suppression | N1 | A1 | B1 | C1 |
| 2. Evidence of moderate suppression | N2 | A2 | B2 | C2 |
| 3. Severe suppression | N3 | A3 | B3 | C3 |

* Children whose HIV infection status is not confirmed are classified by using the above grid with a letter E (for perinatally exposed) placed before the appropriate classification code (e.g., EN2).

Pediatric age group thus requires a specialized attention for diagnosis and therapy. These innocent sufferers have to be dealt with love, affection and expertise to alleviate their untold sufferings.

# 6

# Pathology of AIDS

The pathological features of this acquired immune deficiency may be reflected in various tissues of the body, such as the lymph nodes, thymus, spleen, bone marrow, lymphoid elements of the gastrointestinal tract, testes and kidneys. The morphologic manifestation of infections and neoplasms occurring in AIDS, of course, will also show their own characteristic pathology displayed in the target organs. The opportunistic infections, for example, may affect the central nervous system, gastrointestinal system or the respiratory system, and thus, will cause their specific pathological alterations in these tissues, with demonstration of the causative microbes from within the tissues. In the same way, the bizarre malignancies, such as B-cells lymphomas and Kaposi's sarcomas will display their own histopathologic characteristics. An utmost precaution is, however, required for handling these tissues of the AIDS patient, as they can infect the dealing personnel. For the same reason, caution should be exercised to avoid people who are pregnant, immunosuppressed or have open wounds. Only selected laboratories, well-equipped to deal with such tissues under strict isolation, should be authorised to undertake these procedures. Any direct contact of skin, conjunctiva and mucous membrane should be avoided with the tissues, blood, excretions and body fluids of AIDS patients. Double gloves are recommended, and accidental injuries have to be avoided. The clothes, the face-mask and the goggles worn should be water-proof and disposable, and discarded carefully. The work surfaces, containers and instruments should be decontaminated with 1:10 dilution of 5.25 per cent sodium hypochloride in water for a requisite period of time. Following this, the instruments have to be autoclaved for 45 minutes at 121°C at over 20 pound pressure per square inch. The AIDS-tissues should not be given to random researchers, nor the organs of these patients distributed for transplantation. Enough warning should be affixed on these materials.

## LYMPH NODES

A spectrum of histopathological changes can be discerned in the enlarged lymphnodes of AIDS and pre-AIDS, which can be of a reliable prognostic value in evaluating the time course of progression of the disease. Three patterns of changes can be encountered viz. hyperplasia, partial depletion and burnt-out (Fig. 6.1).

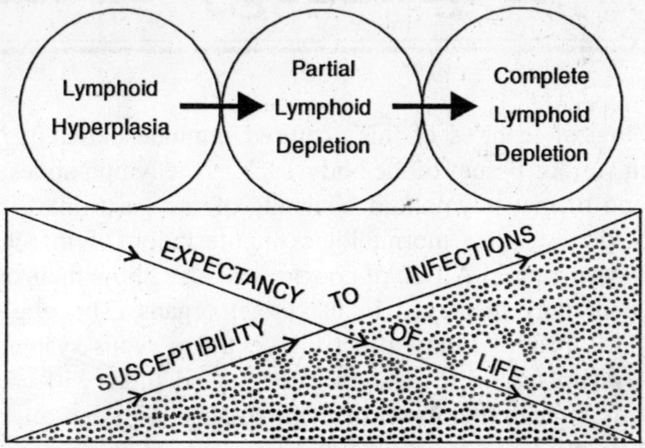


**Fig. 6.1. The Spectrum of Lymphnode Histopathology and its repercussion on host.**

The hyperplastic lymphnodes show a gross enlargement. They are tan, mobile, discrete and soft. The histopathologic features are visible in the form of floridly reactive follicular hyperplasia, with prominent, irregularly-shaped germinal centres undergoing pronounced mitosis, having many tingible body macrophages. The interfollicular areas show an occasional immunoblast (large lymphocyte with vesicular nuclei). There are perivascular clusters of polymorphs and/or plasma cells. Rarely, multinucleated giant cells can also be identified. With the exception of the follicular hyperplasia pattern with follicular fragmentation that is seen most frequently in inguinal and axillary lymph nodes, these patterns appear in lymph nodes throughout the body, regardless of the presence or absence of gross lymph node enlargement, and indicate that a single node biopsy will yield valid findings.

The pattern of follicular hyperplasia gradually transforms to a pattern of partial lymphoid depletion. This is heralded with the gradual loss of paracortical (T-cell area) lymphocytes. The follicular mantles become poorly-defined and gradually lost. There is a variable hyalinization of the germinal centres, often with a prominent interfollicular plasmacytosis. This slowly moulds into a picture of severe to complete lymphoid depletion of both T-and B-cell areas. The lymph node cortex is narrow or undefined and the medulla occupies two thirds or more of the cross-sectional area. Small blood vessels appear prominent due to a decreased overall cellularity, and scattered histiocytes appear in sinuses. Immunoblasts and/or plasma cells may be seen throughout the node. This end stage indicates a very poor prognosis. It may frequently be a finding at the autopsy.

There is a direct correlation of the immunological peripheral-blood-changes with immunohistopathological features of lymphnodes. Immunohistology, however, is distinctly preferable to H&E stained histopathology, as it offers a much greater diagnostic precision in labelling a biopsy as derived from an AIDS or prodromal-AIDS patient. Both the AIDS patients and those with persistent generalized lymphadenopathy display fewer T-helper ($T_4$) cells and a preponderance of T-suppressor/cytotoxic ($T_8$) lymphocytes, when the frozen sections of their lymphnodes are subjected to quantitative T-cell and B-cell immunohistology. Further, an increased number of cells with suppressor T-phenotype can be seen in follicular centres and mantle zone, the B-cell areas. In contrast, the paracortical T-cell areas and germinal centre reveal a distinct paucity of cells with helper T-phenotypes. A depletion of B-lymphocytes is an additional finding of lymphnodes with partial effacement of architecture. Another prominent feature is the intense staining for Ia of the lymphocytes in the interfollicular and medullary sinus areas, even in the prodromal stages.

Lymph node histopathologic changes with HIV infection in children may differ from those in adults. Findings reported at autopsy, mostly in association with deaths from AIDS, have included marked lymphocyte depletion, more selective follicular or paracortical atrophy, hemophagocytosis, hyperplasia, and lymphadenitis. About half of cases with lymphadenitis are due to an identifiable opportunistic infectious agent.

Certain lymphnode findings are specific for opportunistic infections/neoplasms. Massive lymphadenopathy may indicate infection by *Mycobacterium avium* complex (MAC). Mesenteric and retroperitoneal lymphadenopathy demonstrate homogenous soft tissue attenuation by computed tomographic scan. If the involvement is extensive, a grossly lemon-yellow cut surface of lymph node, similar in color to microbiologic culture plates, may be observed. Microscopically, MAC in lymph node is characterized by single cells, small clusters, or large sheets of pale blue striated histiocytes without significant inflammation or necrosis with hematoxylin-eosin staining. Wright-Giemsa stains can give these histiocytes the appearance of Gaucher-like cell. Acid-fast stains will reveal the presence of numerous mycobacteria in the histiocytes.

*Mycobacterium tuberculosis* (MTB) is being seen with increasing frequency as a complication of HIV infection. The sites for involvement with tuberculous lymphadenitis include cervical lymph nodes in virtually all cases, followed by axillary involvement in 82%, ilioinguinal in 54%, and epitrochlear in 36%. The nodal size ranges from 1 to 3 cm, and involvement is usually symmetrical. The presentation overlaps with HIV lymphadenopathy. Histologically, there is usually a recognizable localized granulomatous reaction, including caseous necrosis. Langhans giant cells, lymphocytes, epithelioid histiocytes, and fibrosis are present in variable proportion. Acid-fast tissue stain reveals rod-shaped acid-fast micro-organisms similar to that described in non-HIV-infected patients. The organisms in the lesions are never as numerous with *M tuberculosis* as with MAC.

Lymph node involvement with the dimorphic fungi *C. neoformans, H. capsulatum,* and *C. immitis* is quite frequent as these infections are often disseminated. The lymph nodes may be moderately enlarged and pale or mottled. Visible granulomas are infrequent. Cryptococci appear as clusters of oval, narrow-based budding organisms. The capsule is often missing so that the organism appears small enough to be confused with *Candida* or *H. capsulatum.*

Lymphadenopathy may occasionally occur due to Kaposi's sarcoma (KS), though often there will be no grossly identifiable features. By computed tomographic scan, lymph nodes enlarged by KS may show high attenuation secondary to the increased vascularity of this neoplasm. Involvement of lymph nodes by non-Hodgkin's lymphoma is less frequent than, either central nervous system or gastrointestinal tract. Lymph nodes may be secondarily involved with widespread systemic disease, either with recurrence, or with progression of disease. Multicentric Castleman's disease (MCD) has been occasionally found in persons with HIV infection. Over half of patients with MCD will also have KS. The lesions of MCD with HIV infection appear similar to lesions in non-HIV infected patients. Pathologic findings include small hyalinized germinal centers surrounded by concentric layers of small lymphocytes, vascular hyperplasia, hyalinized vessels, and large sheets of interfollicular plasma cells. Most patients will have a polyclonal gammopathy.

## SPLEEN

Yet another consistent feature of AIDS patients is variable splenomegaly, which, at necropsy, reveal profound congestion, near absence of the germinal centres and a profound lymphoid depletion of T and B-cell areas in histopathological sections. Concomitantly, the evidence of Kaposi's sarcoma may be present. Acute splenitis may also be seen if there has been a disseminated infection. Splenic macrophages studded with the acid-fast bacilli or fungal organisms are the usual feature of acute splenitis. The most frequent splenic findings at autopsy are *M avium* complex (MAC), *M tuberculosis* (MTB), cryptococcosis, cytomegalovirus, Kaposi's sarcoma, and malignant lymphomas.

Gross pathologic lesions consists of a prominent follicular pattern in about half of AIDS cases and a miliary granulomatous pattern in about 10%. Sepsis may lead to a soft, almost liquid spenic parenchyma. Splenic infarcts may occur. At autopsy, young children and infants with HIV infection, most of whom died from AIDS, may show a variety of histologic changes in the spleen. These can include marked lymphocyte depletion of white pulp and hemophagocytosis. In addition, about half of cases may demonstrate so-called "kaposiform" lesions composed of foci with spindle cells admixed with plasma cells, capillaries and hemosiderin laden macrophages.

## BONE MARROW

There may be overall hypercellularity early in the course of AIDS, or with systemic infections, seen in about half to three fourths of cases. This is most often due to hyperplasia of granulocytic or megakaryocytic cell lines. Debilitation leads to increasing hypocellularity and serous atrophy of fat later in the course of AIDS. Additional non-specific microscopic findings may include immature or dysplastic myeloid precursors (dysmyelopoiesis), lymphoid aggregates, atypical megakaryocytes, a fine reticulin fibrosis, mild vascular proliferation, histiocytosis with or without non-specific granuloma formation, and increased hemosiderin deposition. A fairly consistent finding is increased plasma cell cuffing of blood vessels, which may be accompanied by polyclonal hypergammaglobulinemia in over 80% of patients.

Granulomas are infrequently present in bone marrow and may contain fungi, acid-fast organisms, occasional parasites, or polarizable talc crystals from intravenous drug use. These granulomas are typically not well-formed. Localized ill-defined granulomas consisting of collections of histiocytes are more frequent than granulomas containing organisms. Of the dimorphic fungi, *C neoformans* is seen most frequently. *H capsulatum,* next in frequency may produce loose lymphohistiocytic aggregates. Of the mycobacteria, *Mycobacterium avium* complex (MAC) is seen more frequently than *M tuberculosis.* Non-Hodgkin's lymphomas (NHLs) involve the bone marrow in about one fourth of cases in which they are diagnosed at autopsy. Bone marrow biopsy is of value in staging of these lymphomas.

## PERIPHERAL BLOOD

Anemia, thrombocytopenia, neutropenia, lymphocytopenia, monocytopenia, or combinations of any or all of these can occur in over 90% of patients with AIDS. Anemia is present in over half of patients early in the course of AIDS and in nearly all AIDS patients late in the course. The anemia is often normochromic and normocytic, typical of anemia of chronic disease, and iron stores are increased by measurement of serum ferritin. These disorders can be potentiated by zidovudine (ZDV) or trimethoprim-sulfamethoxazole therapy and may require dose reduction or cessation of therapy.

Thrombocytopenia is commonly seen in about a third of AIDS cases, is rarely severe, and may result from peripheral consumption (sphenomegaly, immune complexes) or from decreased marrow platelet production. Lymphopenia is present in about a third of AIDS cases due to the decrease in T4 lymphocytes. Neutropenia can be common in patients with AIDS and is a risk factor for both bacterial and fungal infections. The most common cause for neutropenia is however, drug therapy.

## HEPATOBILIARY SYSTEM

A common clinical and pathologic finding in liver with AIDS is hepatomegaly, seen in about two thirds of cases. Steatosis is a common histopathologic finding. Severe steatosis is a rare but potentially life-threatending complication of antiretroviral therapy with nucleoside reverse transcriptase inhibitors, manifested by lactic acidosis. In pediatric cases, granulomas are less frequent but giant cells more numerous, and lymphoplasmacytic infiltrates can be present in association with lymphocytic interstitial pneumonitis of the lung. Focal fatty change is often present, sometimes with hepatocyte necrosis. Other frequent findings include portal chronic inflammation and fibrosis. Chronic active hepatitis is not seen.

*Mycobacterium avium* complex (MAC) is the most frequent opportunistic infection involving the liver, found in half of AIDS cases with infection with this organism. It produces moderate to marked hepatomegaly. *Mycobacterium tuberculosis* may be seen in liver with dissemination and produces small tan to white granulomas tunlikely to cause hepatomegaly. The dimorphic fungi *C neoformans, H capsulatum,* and *C immitis* involve the liver frequently in disseminated infections, and may be associated with mild abnormalities of liver function tests with hepatomegaly. Cytomegalovirus (CMV) can involve liver in AIDS especially with disseminated infection, rarely causing a mass lesion. Toxoplasma gondii are infrequent and rarely cause a widespreaded infection.

One fifth of Kaposis sarcoma(KS) patients may have liver involvement. Microscopically, KS may show dilated vascular spaces similar to hemangioma, but hemangiomas will not have atypical spindle cells. Non-Hodgkin's lymphoma (NHL) may appear in liver in association with widespread dissemination and only rarely as a primary tumor. Persistent fever, tender hepatomegaly, mildly abnormal liver function tests and an elevated lactate dehydrogenase are typical clinical findings. Around 70% to 90% of persons with a history of intravenous drug use have serologic evidence for hepatitis B virus (HBV) infection, and up to 10 or 20% of all patients with HIV infection can have chronic HBV infection. HIV infection appears to be associated with increased viral replication and a greater carriage rate for HBV than in non-HIV-infected patients.

Hepatotoxicity can appear in the course of AIDS in patients treated with a variety of pharmacologic agents. Half of patients receiving prophylaxis for *Pneumocystis carinii* with either trimethoprim-sulfamethoxazole (TMP-SMX) or pentamidine have elevations in transaminases or alkaline phosphatase but severe hepatotoxicity is uncommon. Sulfa drugs can also cause a granulomatous hepatitis. Both ketoconazole and fluconazole used to treat fungal infections can be associated with transaminase elevations in 10 to 20% of cases. Agents used to treat *Mycobacterium tuberculosis,* such as isoniazid and rifampin, can produce enough abnormalities in liver function tests to alter the therapeutic regimen in 5% of cases. The antiretroviral agent didanosine (ddI) is associated with transaminase elevations in one third of treated patients.

The biliary tract and gallbladder may occasionally be involved by a variety of lesions including acalculous cholecystitis, sclerosing cholangitis, and papillary stenosis. Collectively, these lesions are known as AIDS cholangiopathy, and most patients who exhibit these findings have a CD4 count <200/microliter. AIDS cholangiopathy may manifest as a secondary sclerosing cholangitis with epigastric pain, fever, diarrhea, and increased alkaline phosphatase. The bilirubin may not be elevated.

## CARDIOVASCULAR SYSTEM

Heart is not a conventional site for opportunistic infection or neoplasm. A congestive (dilated) cardiomyopathy in both adult and pediatric AIDS patients has been identified in 10 to 30% of cases. Most of these cases are idiopathic, for no specific opportunistic infection or neoplasm can be identified. A non-specific myocarditis composed mainly of mononuclear cells appears, more commonly than infectious organisms in the heart of AIDS patients. Pericardial effusions may be seen in about 40% of persons with HIV infection. In most of these cases, the effusion is small and clinically insignificant. A specific etiology for the effusion, which can include a variety of infectious agents, is found in about a fourth of cases.

A high grade non-Hodgkin's lymphoma is the commonest AIDS diagnostic disease seen in heart, occurring in about one sixth of AIDS cases. The lymphoma is usually diagnosed at autopsy.

## RESPIRATORY TRACT

Respiratory tract diseases account for one half deaths from AIDS. The pathology of respiratory tract conforms to the causative opportunistic infection or the neoplasm, and are dealt with in respective chapters on infections and neoplasms.

*Pneumocystis* is more likely to have a diffuse involvement of lung than other opportunistic infectious agents or neoplasms with AIDS. It typically involves alveolar spaces, giving the gross appearance of pneumonic consolidation. *Pneumocystis carinii* pneumonia (PCP) tends to be more confluent throughout the lungs than bacterial pneumonias. Cut surfaces of lung with early PCP show a prominent "poached salmon" or pale pink appearance when in the fresh state, and the markedly consolidated lung is firm to friable with a definable lobular pattern with scattered areas of hemorrhage or congestion.

*Mycobacterium tuberculosis* will usually produce grossly recognizable tan to white firm granulomas, often with caseation. Sometimes, the granulomas involve the pleura and are associated with a hemorrhagic exudate or effusion. Microscopically, the classical features of caseation with Langhans giant cells, fibrosis, and lymphocytic infiltration are present but not pronounced. In acid fast stains, mycobacteria are scattered singly or in small clusters, numerous and easy to demonstrate.

In AIDS, toxoplasmosis is usually associated with disseminated infection and secondary pulmonary involvement. An abnormal chest roentgenogram marked by bilateral interstitial infiltrates may appear in only half of cases. Diagnosis can be made by bronchoalveo-lavage in most cases. Histologically, there may be focal necrosis with vague granuloma formation and/or diffuse interstitial mixed inflammatory cell infiltrates with alveolar lining cell hyperplasia. Diagnosis depends upon finding *Toxoplasma gondii* pseudocysts filled with bradyzoites, but these are infrequent – even in severe infections.

## CENTRAL NERVOUS SYSTEM

HIV encephalopathy is associated with a progressive debilitating dementia. Examination of cerebrospinal fluid (CSF) reveal no specific findings. Radiological feature include a diffuse cortical atrophy and deep white matter abnormalities. Both neuron and glial cells are not directly infected with HIV. Instead, the CNS damage is mediated through infection of phagocytic cells – macrophages and microglial cells – that are infected with HIV. The phagocytic cells release cytokines and viral factors that lead to neuronal damage and dropout. HIV leukoencephalopathy may be seen in about 5% of AIDS patients at autopsy. It produces diffuse bilateral damage to cerebral white matter that can be seen on magnetic resonance imaging (MRI). Occasionally, the cerebellum is also involved. There is myelin loss involving mainly the deep white matter, with a tendency to spare the subcortical U fibers and the more compact myelin bundles of corpus callosum, internal capsules, optic radiations, and descending tracts in the brainstem.

HIV infection producing a myelitis is present in only about 8% of AIDS cases. Vacuolar myelopathy of the spinal cord may be seen in only one third of AIDS cases, and though it is probably a consequence of HIV infection, it is not usually associated with HIV mayelitis. It is manifested only when vacuolization is severe, and presents with slowly progressive spastic paraparesis accompanied by loss of vibratory and position sense and urinary frequency/urgency. Toxoplasmosis, malignant lymphomas, cryptococcosis, and cytomegalovirus are the most commonly identified opportunistic infections and neoplasms in the CNS in patients with AIDS.

## GASTROINTESTINAL TRACT

The gastrointestinal (GI) tract is the second most common organ system site for opportunistic infections or neoplasms associated with AIDS. Oral candidiasis, (thrush) is a frequent finding in patients with HIV infection that precedes or accompanies clinical AIDS. The risk for development of oral thrush is increased with smoking.

Radiologic findings in association with esophageal candidiasis include discreet linear or irregular longitudinally oriented filling defects that represent the heaped-up mucosal plaques. Esophagography may reveal a markedly irregular, shaggy mucosal appearance with more advanced esophageal disease. Other infecting organisms too attack the GI tract with variable frequency. The GI tract is one of the most common sites of involvement by non-Hodgkin's lymphomas (NHL) in patients with AIDS. These lymphomas occur most frequently in the stomach, small intestine, and colon. Unlike Kaposi's sarcoma, gastrointestinal lymphomas may be symptomatic from complications of obstruction, perforation, or bleeding. Similarly, Kaposi sarcoma involves gastrointestinal tract most commonly after the skin.

## ENDOCRINE ORGAN PATHOLOGY

Most opportunistic infections and neoplasms affecting the endocrine system in patients with AIDS occur when these diseases are widely disseminated. The most common endocrine organ affected is the adrenal gland. Adrenal involvement with other opportunistic infections and neoplasms usually occurs with widespread dissemination and is only diagnosed at autopsy. Grossly, lesions of the adrenal are difficult to detect. Marked adrenal enlargement from any opportunistic infection is not common. Malignant lymphomas can, occasionally cause unilateral or bilateral enlargement with white-tan to red variegated masses or infiltrates. Cytomegalovirus may produce a multifocal reddish mottling within the yellow cortex. Kaposi's sarcoma may infiltrate the periadrenal fat or the substance of the gland in a linear dark-red to purple pattern.

Thyroid and Parathyroid glands can only occasionally be involved by cytomegalovirus, *Pneumocytis carinii* or dimorphus fungi in their disseminated form, as is the case with Pituitary gland.

## GENITO URINARY SYSTEM

The male genital tract has no specific pathologic changes resulting from HIV infection despite the fact seminal fluid is a common vehicle for transmission of HIV. By in situ hybridization, HIV-1 proviral DNA can be identified within the germ cells at all stages of differentiation but without morphologic changes. The testis in AIDS shows an atropy somewhat like that of chronic alcoholism. There is decreased or absent spermatogenesis, peritubular fibrosis and loss of germ cells – but opportunistic infections and neoplasms are rare. Prostate and seminal vesicle are occasionally the site for KS and CMV when these are widely disseminated. One important finding in prostate is cryptococcal prostatitis seen with disseminated cryptococcosis.

Women with HIV infection are more likely to have concomitant human papillomavirus (HPV) infection and have a subsequent higher risk for high grade cervical intraepithelial neoplasia (CIN) and invasive cervical squamous cell carcinomas. The rate of cervical squamous intraepithelial lesions (SILs) in HIV infected women is 4.5 times that of uninfected women, and 1 in 5 HIV-infected women with an apparently normal cervix will develop a SIL within 3 years.

The kidney may show a so-called "HIV-associated nephropathy" (HIVAN), or HIV nephropathy (HIVN). About 50% of persons developing HIVAN have a history of injection drug use. In over 90%, the affected person is Black, though a few are Hispanic, and the disease is rare in Caucasians. HIVAN is characterized by marked proteinuria and a rapid progression to renal failure and end stage renal disease (ESRD). Patients are typically normotensive. Rising serum urea nitrogen and creatinine levels in a non-terminal patient may suggest nephropathy. For diagnosis of HIVAN, total protein excretion should exceed 100 mg/m$^2$ in a child or 200-500 mg in an adult.

The kidneys with HIVAN can be grossly enlarged (10 to 25%), appearing echogenic by ultrasound. However, they do not become atrophic, even in the later stages. The most common renal biopsy finding, seen in over 80% of cases, is focal segmental glomerulosclerosis (FSGS). Diffuse mesangial hypercellularity is the most common pattern seen in children.

## OPHTHALMIC PATHOLOGY

Cytomegalovirus is the most common clinical and autopsy ocular finding in patients with AIDS. CMV retinitis may be seen in 30 to 40% of AIDS patients at some point in their course. This infection is most likely to occur when the CD4 count is below 100/microliter. Cytomegalovirus can be confirmed at autopsy by finding characteristic inclusion bodies in the choroid. About half of CMV retinitis cases have an acute inflammatory reaction.

The second most common cause for retinitis in AIDS is infection with the Varicella-zoster virus (VZV), seen in 1 to 4% of HIV-infected persons, typically when there is involvement of the ophthalmic division of the trigeminal nerve.

A non-infective retinal microvasculopathy of unknown origin is also observed in half of AIDS patients.

## ELECTRON MICROSCOPIC FEATURES

The ultrastructural observation of AIDS tissues, lymphoreticular elements in particular, reveal certain interesting inclusion bodies. The etiologic HIV-1 viral inclusion is seen as 100 to 120 nm inclusion. Then, there are test-tube and ring-shaped inclusions, seen within the lymphocytes as concentrically arranged endoplasmic reticulum cisternae, with electron-dense material interposed in the cytosol between layers. Tubuloreticular inclusions may also be seen, and are subcellular organelles composed of nuclease and RNA-resistant complexes of lipid-rich membranes, and proteins composed of fine tubular meshwork, developing within and distending the endoplasmic reticulum. They are thought to be related to viral infections and autoimmune phenomenon. Another type of inclusion bodies observed in the AIDS patients are the vesicular rosettes, located in the cytoplasm of lymphoid cells of lymphnodes. They are formed by numerous 30 to 60 nm vesicles radially clustered around an electron dense core. As they can also be sporadically detected in the control group, they best represent an expression of some degenerative changes.

## HISTOPATHOLOGY OF MALIGNANCIES

Kaposi's sarcoma, as will be discussed elsewhere, is the commonest neoplasm developing in AIDS. This has been classified by Krigel and his associates into 4 clinically distinct forms as (a) cutaneous, locally indolent, seen in elderly, (b) cutaneous, locally aggressive with/without regional lymphnode enlargement, seen in Africa, (c) generalized mucocutaneous or lymphadenopathic disease, and (d) disseminated mucocutaneous or lymphadenopathic disease, and (d) disseminated mucocutaneous disease with visceral involvement. Of the 4 types, AIDS patients develop (c) type of disease, exhibiting as fulminant angioproliferative disorder of the endothelial origin. The endothelial cells have factor VIII related antigen as one of the prominent markers. The electron microscopy reveals the presence of rod-shaped cytoplasmic organelles, the Weibal-Palade bodies, in these cells. However, they can also be demonstrated in non-AIDS Kaposi's sarcoma. The Kaposi's sarcoma in AIDS, by virtue of its pattern of dissemination suggests a multicentric origin rather than haematogenous metastatic spread. Lymphnodes are commonly affected, and exhibit haemorrhagic lesions in capsular, subcapsular, sinusoidal and hilar location. Visceral lesions are equally common.

The gross examination of visceral lesions display a haemorrhagic look, arising in association with the blood vessels such as epicardial coronary arteries in heart, portal tract in liver, and so on. In lungs, they appear as erythematous nodules and plaques in approximation to pleura, perivascular location, along bronchus and interlobular septae. It may be accompanied by serosanguinous pleural effusion. In advanced stages, it may cause massive intra-alveolar haemorrahages resulting in death. The macroscopic appearance of gastrointestinal lesions reveals a flat nodulo-vascular character, originating in the submucosa and extending to lamina propria, producing mucosal ulcerations.

Microscopic pathology of Kaposi's sarcoma can conveniently be classified as 'angiomatous', 'classic' and 'sarcomatous', extending as a continuous spectrum. The usual features include arrangement of neoplastic cells into slit-like vascular spaces, proliferating spindle-shaped cells, scattered red-blood cells, haemosiderin deposits, collections of plasma cells, few mitotic figures, mild nuclear atypia and characteristic PAS-positive, diastase-resistant intracellular hyaline globules. The histo-pathological differential diagnosis includes dermatofibroma, pyogenic granuloma, stasis dermatitis, telengiectasia, angiosarcoma and florid granulation tissue. The lesions in the integument characteristically dissect through collagen of the mid-dermis, exhibiting a prediliction for perivascular areas. The electron microscopic appearance of small blood vessels of Kaposi's sarcoma demonstrate a lack of prominent investment of pericytes and their processes, absent/fragmentory basal lamina, and discontinuity in the endothelial linings.

The AIDS-related lymphomas are usually of non-Hodgkin's type, and seen most frequently in the central nervous system. The other common sites are the abdomen, oropharynx, jaws, rectum, orbit, lymphnodes, kidneys, muscles, liver and the bone marrow. They are quite unpredictable, and may either remain localized or spread far and wide. They are characteristically diffuse in architecture. Histopathologically, they are small, non-cleaved (undifferentiated) or large cell (histiocytic) subtypes. The high rate of cellular turnover, particularly in undifferentiated variety, displays a starry sky's pattern. Hodgkin's lymphomas have also been recorded in AIDS patients.

## IMMUNOLOGICAL PROFILE

It is now well-established that the causative virus of AIDS attacks predominantly the $T_4$ lymphocytes, and from there ensures a serious imbalance of the cell-mediated immune functions of the body. In this process, several immunologic abnormalities, which may, well, be characteristic enough for the certain diagnosis of AIDS, are produced. The humoral responses, too, are affected in the process. The common immunologic aberrations observed in AIDS and pre-AIDS are enumerated in the table 6.1.

**Table 6.1: Immunological Aberrations of AIDS and Pre-AIDS**

**Aberrations of cell-mediated immunity:**

- lymphocytopenia
- T-lymphocyte dysfunction
- $T_4$-depletion ($CD_4$, Helper/inducer lymphocytes)
- $T_4 : T_8$ ratio alteration ($CD_4 : CD_8$ ratio inversion)
- Defective response to mitogens and antigens
- Thymic involution and epithelial destruction

**Aberrations of humoral immunity:**

- Spontaneous B-cell proliferation and differentiation.
- Decreased B-cell response to mitogens.
- Lack of *de novo* antigen response.
- Circulating acid-labile alpha interferon and immune complexes (CIC)
- Non-specific anti-lymphocyte antibodies.
- Elevated alpha-1 thymosin levels.
- Defects in monocyte functions.
- Elevated beta-2 microglobulin levels.
- Decreased serum-thymulin levels.
- Increased soluble interleukin-2 receptor level
- Presence of circulating and inducible suppressor factors.

## Immunologic abnormalities in AIDS-related complex (ARC)

AIDS-related complex, as discussed elsewhere, includes those high-risk patients exposed and infected with HIV-1 virus, and having signs and symptoms related to AIDS, yet not fulfilling all the criteria of the Centres for Disease Control. The usual immunological abnormalities that can be recorded in these subjects are cutaneous anergy, decreased non-killer (NK) cell activity, impaired responsiveness to both T-cell and B-cell mitogens, and serologic evidence of HIV-1 exposure. Not all patients of ARC develop AIDS, even after many years following exposure. Subsequent development of AIDS is usually associated with a gradually deteriorating cellular immune functions, as measured by the standard immunologic tests.

## Immunologic abnormalities in full-blown AIDS

The preliminary observations of this novel syndrome recording severe depletion of both number and functions of $T_4$ (helper/inducer) lymphocytes, suggested a lymphocytotropic agent which selectively assaulted these cells. This was later designated as HTLV-III or HIV-1. This virus has a specific tropism for the $T_4$-lymphocytes, and from their interaction, a host of immunological distortions gradually emerge. This virus has an additional potential of altering normal functions of $T_8$-lymphocytes, NK cells, monocytes and B-lymphocytes.

T-lymphocyte dysfunctions have been the most salient as well as crucial abnormalities perceptible in the HIV-1 infections culminating in full-blown AIDS. Lymphocytopenia has been a consistent finding, which in advanced stages of infection may become lower than 500/cu mm. The brunt of the disease, however, is chiefly borne by the cells bearing the helper/inducer phenotype ($OKT_4$) i.e $T_4$-lymphocytes, resulting in an apparent excess of $CD_8$ (cytotoxic/supressor) lymphocytes, and thus a lowered $CD_4$: $CD_8$ ratio. Further, the $CD_4$-lymphocyte count has been found to be significantly lower in patients with opportunistic infections than those with Kaposi's sarcoma or other malignancies. As opportunistic infections form a bad prognostic marker of AIDS, in analogy, a decreasing $T_4$-lymphocyte count is directly proportional to a worsening prognosis.

Although, delayed hypersensitivity is usually intact early in the syndrome, yet, as the disease progresses, there is an increasing cutaneous anergy to the standard test antigens. The development of protozoal, viral, fungal and bacterial infections, as well as that of bizarre malignancies reflect a disorganised/shattered T-lymphocyte function. The same scenario is reflected *in vitro* as well, in the form of a defective response to T-cell mitogens and also an aberrant cytotoxic and mixed lymphocyte response. In addition, there is an alteration in the production of lymphokines by the T-cells and a diminished helper function (for B-cell immunoglobulin production). A defective auto and allo-reactive responses have also been recorded in bulk T-cell cultures of AIDS patients. So is the lymphokine production by them. Mononuclear cells derived from these patients, demonstrate an impaired mitogen-induced gamma interferon production, which may practically be absent in response to invading microbes.

B-lymphocyte dysfunction is yet another complement in AIDS patients, manifesting as elevated serum immunoglobulin levels, demonstration of immune complexes, and exhibiting autoimmune phenomenon. *In vitro* studies reveal that AIDS patients have a significant number of spontaneous plaque-forming cells in their peripheral blood than the healthy controls, thus demonstrating an increased number of B-cells, spontaneously secreting immunoglobulins IgG and IgA. A serious handicap in the normal proliferation of B-cells to T-cells dependent B-cell mitogen, poke-weed mitogen or to T-cell independent mitogen (*Staphylococcus aureus* Cowan-1) results from the defective $T_4$-cell number and function. The crux thus, elaborate that B-cells from AIDS patients are pre-activated, proliferating and secreting immunoglobulins, but incapable of responding to signals that normally trigger resting B-cells.

Monocyte functions are also abnormal in AIDS, and are reflected in the form of defective chemotaxis and ineffective extracellular killing of the parasites. Further, they do not produce interleukin-1, should such a stimulus occur. Akin to the B-lymphocyte profile, AIDS monocytes are also in a preactivated state, causing spontaneous secretion of interleukin-1 and prostaglandin $E_2$, but failing utterly when need arises.

Another significant immunological feature of AIDS patients is aberration of both NK-cell activity and T-cell mediated cytotoxicity against infected target cells, manifesting as a markedly decreased NK lysis of tumour cells, and a decreased specific killing of target cells infected with cytomegalovirus respectively. *In vitro*, these abnormalities revert back to normal should purified interleukin-2 is added to the culture of AIDS-lymphocytes.

The sera of AIDS-patients also show certain alterations, which are recounted in table 6.2.

**Table 6.2: Serological alteration in AIDS**

1. Elevation of alpha-1 thymosin
2. Elevation of beta-2 microglobulin
3. Presence of acid-labile alpha interferon
4. Demonstration of suppressive factors
5. Demonstration of anti-lymphocyte antibodies
6. Decreased serum thymulin levels

The salient laboratory abnormalities, thus include anaemia, leukopenia, lymphopenia and thrombocytopenia, but an apparently normal bone-marrow. Liver enzymes may be slightly raised, but kidney functions are usually normal. A rapid deterioration of kidney functions may be a feature of focal/segmental glomerulosclerosis. Further, raised immunoglobulin levels are present, where IgG is usually over 2000 mg/dl and IgA over 350 mg/dl. IgM ordinarily remains unaltered. Cutaneous anergy to standard test antigens is another feature, as is the presence of the immune complexes. The diagnostic hallmark of AIDS, however, is selective depletion of the $CD_4$ lymphocytes.

# 7

# Spectrum of Infections

The acquired immunodeficiency syndrome predisposes the affected individual extremely susceptible for the development of bizarre and unusually extensive infections, as the quantum of immunodeficiency progresses. The malignancy originating in AIDS patients is seldom the cause of death, as it takes a relatively longer time to prove fatal. The infection, on the other hand, is the prime killer of these patients, as it becomes exceptionally florid in a matter of days or weeks in full-blown-AIDS patients, and rapidly causes multi-system failure and death. Moreover, the etiologic agents of such infections are the microbes who seldom affect a normal human being, ordinarily inhabiting as saprophytes in the environment. For the same reason, there are not many drugs and/or vaccines hitherto worked out for them. These invading organisms of AIDS patients are unique, (Table 7.1) for they seldom are encountered in other immunodeficiency states.

**Table 7.1: Common opportunistic infections (OI) in AIDS**

| Group | Organisms |
|---|---|
| Protozoa | *Pneumocystis carinii* • *Taxoplasma gondii*<br>*Cryptospordium sp.* |
| Fungi | *Candida sp.* • *Cryptococcus neoformans* |
| Bacteria | *M. tuberculosis* • *Legionella sp.*<br>*M. avium-intercellulare* |
| Viruses | *Cytomegalovirus* • *Herpes simplex*<br>*Herpes zoster* • *Hepatitis virus*<br>*Epstein-Barr virus* |

The incidence and type of the opportunistic infection seen in AIDS in often linked to the CD4+ count in the HIV infected patient (table 7.2). With the institution of highly active antiretroviral therapy (HAART) there is some decline in the incidence of opportunistic infections. Individual organisms have different incidence and thus have to be kept in mind where ever some suspicion arises.

**Table 7.2: Correlation of opportunistic infections with CD4 Cell Counts**

| CD4 cell count | Opportunistic infections |
|---|---|
| **CD4 cell count > 500/mm³** | |
| | Acute retroviral syndrome |
| | Candidial vaginitis |
| **CD4 cell count > 200 - 500/mm³** | |
| | Pneumococcal and other bacterial pneumonias |
| | Pulmonary TB |
| | Herpes zoster |
| | Thrush (Candidiasis) |
| | Candidial esophagitis |
| | Cryptosporidiosis (self-limited) |
| | Oral hairy leukoplakia |
| | (Kaposi's Sarcoma) |
| **CD4 cell count < 200/mm³** | |
| | *P. carinii* pneumonia |
| | Disseminated/chronic *Herpes simplex* |
| | Toxoplasmosis |
| | Cryptococcosis |
| | Disseminated histoplasmosis and Coccidioidomycosis |
| | Cryptosporidiosis (chronic) |
| | Microsporidiosis |
| | Miliary/extrapulmonary TB |
| | Progressive multifocal leukoencephalopathy (PML) |
| | Candidial esophagitis |
| **CD4 cell count < 50/mm³** | |
| | Disseminated cytomegalovirus infection |
| | Disseminated *M. avium* complex |

The *Pneumocystis carinii* infection, for example, has about 35% to 70% annual attack rate in AIDS patients, while in cancer and organ-transplant patients, this rate is only 0.01 to 1%. In the same context, the organ transplant recipients, patients with haematologic malignancies, and those on immunosuppressives including corticosteroids, commonly get invaded by *Listeria monocytogenes,* which only exceptionally attacks AIDS patient, even in its full-blown stage.

The clinical picture may vary in individual infections, although many organisms may cause similar signs and symptoms. The commonest presentation is the affliction of the respiratory system, followed by other systems such as the gastrointestinal and central nervous system.

## COMMON DISORDERS

### Pneumonia

The involvement of the pulmonary tissue by the infective process can either be an indolent or an acute one. However, the atypical opportunistic infections are usually not suspected, and thus the condition keeps on flaring up in spite of the usual antibiotic therapy, and eventually takes a serious turn. The gravity of the situation warrants a high degree of suspicion, undertaking instant laboratory procedures including isolation of the organisms, and vigorous treatment. The usual clinical features include a variable cough and dyspnoea. The skiagram of the chest is often deceptive, and may be normal or near-normal, as are the arterial blood gases, thus necessitating a diagnostic bronchoscopy. Gallium scans can also be undertaken. A pneumonitis can be anticipated, if the gallium scan shows a diffuse pulmonary uptake which is greater than soft tissue uptake.

The commonest cause of extensive pneumonitis is *P. Carinii,* followed by cytomegalovirus. *C. neoformans*, Kaposi's sarcoma, mycobacteria and other atypical forms. *Pneumocystis carinii* pneumonia (PCP) is the most severe opportunistic infection in patients was AIDS. Over half of all AIDS patients will have at least one episode of PCP at some point during their clinical course, with mortality from a single episode ranging from 10 to 30%. However, use of antipneumocystis therapy and prophylaxis, either with trimethoprim-sulfamethoxazole, dapsone, or aerosolized pentamidine can greatly diminish the incidence of PCP and increase survival. Clinical features of PCP include the classic triad of fever, non-productive cough, and dyspnea. A pleuritic type of chest pain and pleural effusion may be present. Spontaneous pneumothorax is an uncommon complication that can recur and is difficult to treat. PCP may reveal a diffuse homogeneous/patchy nonhomogeneous picture on radiological examination, while nodular/linear infilterates with adenopathy/effusion indicate a Kaposi's sarcoma or a fungal infection. Both the preceding features can occur in one patient.

The sputum and blood cultures may prove rewarding in a percentage of patients. In a sizeable majority, however, fibre-optic bronchoscopy with transbronchial biopsy should be undertaken, when the preceding investigations prove unfruitful. Care should be taken in case the patient suffers from coagulopathies, or cannot be oxygenated adequately with 100 per cent oxygen and no positive pressure.

**Table 7.3: Potential Causes of Respiratory Symptoms in HIV-infected Adults**

| Frequency | Infectious Causes | Noninfectious Causes |
|---|---|---|
| Common | Bacterial pneumonia<br>*Mycobacterium tuberculosis*<br>*Pneumocystis carinii*<br>Respiratory viruses<br>*Cryptococcus neoformans*<br>Endemic mycoses<br>*(e.g. Histoplasma capsulatum, Caccidiodes immitis)* | Nonspecific interstitial pneumonitis |
| Uncommon | Atypical mycobacteria<br>*e.g. Mycobacterium avium complex*<br>*Toxoplasma gondii*<br>*Rhodococcus equi*<br>*Aspergillus spp.*<br>Cytomegalovirus | Lymphoma<br>Pulmonary embolism<br>Congestive heart failure |
| Rare | *Salmonella*<br>Syphilis<br>*Mycobacterium malmoense*<br>*Cryptosporidium*<br>*Strongyloides stercoralis* | Lymphocytic interstitial pneumonitis<br>Talcosis<br>Kaposi's sarcoma |

Tuberculosis is another significant finding in AIDS patients. Worldwide, the reported prevalence of TB in AIDS patients ranges from 4% to 44% in different populations. Compared to non-HIV-infected patients, HIV/TB-infected patients have higher rates of primary disease (37%/6 months vs. 5%/2 years), reactivation disease (7-10%/year vs. 5-8%/lifetime), skin test anergy, and extrapulmonary TB (50%). TB may influence the natural history of HIV by activating macrophages leading to increased HIV expression and rapid progression to AIDS if latent TB is untreated. Overall, patients with a higher $CD_4$ count often present in 'classic" fashion whereas those with low $CD_4$ count are more likely to present atypically. Mycobacterium avium – intercellulare is frequently found in sputum and may sometimes cause invasive pulmonary disease. The potential causes of respiratory symptom are depicted in the table 7.3.

## Central Nervous System affliction

CNS-pathologic lesions are one of the most frequent manifestations of AIDS, and one or more pathologic findings are typically identified in over 80% of autopsied AIDS patients. Of AIDS-diagnostic diseases, cryptococcosis, cytomegalovirus, malignant lymphomas, and toxoplamosis are by far the most frequent. About one-fifth of AIDS patients die from CNS diseases. Focal neurological lesions are not unusual finding in AIDS patients, and manifest as seizures, cognitive disorders or focal sensory and motor deficits. In 10 to 20 per cent AIDS patients, opportunistic infections can gain access to the central nervous system. Lumbar puncture may or may not be of any help. A CT scan may, however, give certain valuable clues. If it shows any contrast-enhancing lesion (s), toxoplasmosis, lymphoma, tuberculoma or cryptococcoma may be the likely diagnosis. In cases where multiple hypodense lesions are present, a progressive multifocal encephalopathy may be anticipated. A brain biopsy of accessible lesions is indicated, but seldom shows a specific pathologic picture. Some patients may present as cryptococcal meningitis. Disseminated zoster and other viral infections may be associated with meningoencephalitis, with multiple cranial nerve abnormalities.

The prevalence of AIDS dementia complex (ADC), or human immunodeficiency virus-associated dementia (HIVD) varies widely. ADC can occur at any stage of HIV infection. During the asymptomatic stage of HIV infection, ADC has been estimated to have an incidence of 0.4%. In 3% of adults with HIV infection, ADC the first manifestation of AIDS. During the late stages of AIDS, when $CD_4$ lymphocyte counts drop and HIV-1 RNA levels increase, more patients may be affected, with up to 30% exhibiting some degree of cognitive impairment and up to 15% developing frank dementia. In patients receiving highly active antiretroviral therapy (HAART) the incidence declines. The disease often progresses insidiously, particularly in patients receiving antiretroviral therapy, but the onset can be more rapid over weeks in patients who have never received antiretroviral therapy. Persons with $CD_4$ counts below 100/ microliter progress more rapidly. The mean survival in untreated persons is about 6 months.

## Fever

There are many causes of fever in AIDS patients, in addition to those affecting normal population. Fever may be a result of infections, malignancies, or due to drug therapy. It is quite a taxing thing to decide for certain the exact cause of fever in AIDS patients, as several causes might be operating together. A battery of investigations is usually needed to identify the cause of fever. It is however, recommended to undertake only the procedures which will identify those underlying causes that are amenable to treatment such as Pneumocystis carinii, and so on. It is no use wasting time in isolating cytomegalovirus or other organism for which no therapy is currently available. The usual tests include blood culture for relevant pathogens, serum cryptococcal antigen, urine, sputum and stool culture for bacteria and protozoa, lymph node biospy, lumbar puncture, CT scan abdomen, and gallium scan. A careful history, sequence of events and a thorough clinical evaluation cannot be overlooked, as it may often give clue to the etiology of fever.

## Gastrointestinal affliction

The most frequent clinical symptom resulting from Gl involvement is diarrhea, and the etiologies for this are numerous. Diarrhea may appear with acute HIV infection, but typically it is manifested in patients with clinical AIDS.

Pathogens that involve the small intestine produce large volume watery stools (up to 10L/day), abdominal cramping, bloating, gas, and weight loss with wasting syndrome. Malabsorbtion can lead to vitamin and other nutrient deficiencies. Bacterial pathogens involving the colon most often produce frequent but small volume stools with painful defecation. Fever is often present. The stools can be bloody or mucoid with leukocytosis, typical for a colitis. Stool culture provides a definitive diagnosis.

The dimorphic fungi *Cryptococcus neoformans, Histoplasma capsulatum,* and *Coccidioides immitis* may produce focal inflammation. The GI tract is usually involved only when there is widespread dissemination. These organisms are most likely to be found in the submucosa or mucosa. Grossly visible features of gastrointestinal histoplasmosis include mucosal ulceration, nodules, and hemorrhage. *Candida* esophagitis is another common GI tract manifestation of AIDS in both adults and children, and patients with oral and esophageal candidiasis usually present with odynophagia and/or dysphagia.

The gastrointestinal tract is the second most common site for KS and the commonest visceral site. In most cases, the GI tract is involved in addition to the skin and/or lymph nodes. Lesions may occur anywhere from the oral cavity to the anus. Grossly, the lesions are raised dark red nodules averaging 0.5 to 1.5 cm in diameter widely scattered, but they may also involve large areas of the mucosal surface. Though the lesions are quite vascular, large hemorrhages are uncommon.

Gastrointestinal protozoal infections in patients with AIDS are not rare. They can be asymptomatic, but the most common symptom is diarrhea. They are transmitted via a fecal-oral route. Cryptosporidiosis is a chronic infection in about half of affected AIDS patients, transient in about one fourth, and fulminant in less than 10%. It is estimated to afflict 10 to 20% of patients of AIDS with diarrhea in the U.S., and half of such patients in developing nations. Cryptosporidiosis produces a voluminous, watery diarrhea with 6 to 25 bowel movements per day with a stool volume of 1 to 17 liters. It is often accompanied by abdominal cramps, low-grade fever, anorexia, electrolyte imbalance, dehydration, and weight loss, though it rarely leads to death. Besides the usual opportunistic infections, other bacterial infections can occur in association with HIV infection. Enteric bacterial infections usually produce stools that do not contain occult blood or leukocytes. Definitive diagnosis is made by stool culture.

Both *Mycobacterium avium*-complex (MAC) and *Mycobacterium tuberculosis* (MTB) are usually found in the small intestine, particularly the duodenum, but can also be found in the colon and stomach. *Mycobacterium tuberculosis* in the GI tract is distributed primarily as small granulomas in cases with widespread dissemination. The most common site of involvement for MTB is the ileocecal region. Colonic lesions are seen radiographically to consist of segmental ulcerations, inflammatory strictures, or hypertrophic lesions resembling polyps.

Cytomegalovrirus (CMV) is capable of infecting all parts of the gastrointestinal tract, but the most common clinical manifestation is colitis. At least 20% of patients with AIDS have gastrointestinal involvement with CMV. Clinically, there may be diarrhea, fever, abdominal pain, hemotachezia, weight loss, or anorexia. Odynophagia would suggest esophageal involvement. There is no typical identifiable pattern of involvement. Gross lesions are often not present, but anything from mucosal erythema to small mucosal ulcers to plaques may occur.

## Oral Cavity Changes

A fourth to half of all persons infected with HIV will have one or more oral lesions during the course of their infection, and in 10% an oral lesion will be the first manifestation of their illness. The most common lesions are oral candidiasis, hairy leukoplakia, periodontitis, gingivitis, aphthous ulcers, and Kaposi's sarcoma. Symptoms may include xerostomia and burning mouth syndrome. Oral papules and ulcers may appear on buccal mocosa with *Histoplasma capsulatum* and *Penicillium marneffei* infections. Hairy leukoplakia, also known as oral condyloma planum, produces a white lesion usually found on the lateral border of the tongue that is slightly raised, poorly demarcated and variable in size. The mucosal surface is grossly corrugated or "hairy". Unlike the exudate of oral thrush, the lesion of hairy leukoplakia cannot be scraped off. Both Epstein-Barr virus (EBV) and papillomavirus have been identified in epithelial cells with hairy leukoplakia. Microscopically, the squamous epithelium shows marked acanthosis (which produces the grossly "hairy" appearance) with parakeratosis, koilocytosis, and herpetic type intranuclear inclusions.

## Anorectal Squamous Intraepithelial Lesions (ASIL)

Persons with HIV infection may develop ASIL that can progress from high-grade squamous intraepithelial lesions (HSIL) to invasive carcinomas. The relative risk for anal intraepithelial lesions is 60 in men and 7.8 in women, compared with persons not infected with HIV. Anorectal squamous cell dysplasia, carcinoma, and condyloma acuminatum all have a higher incidence (7%) in young homosexual males than in the general population, and this incidence is even greater (36%) in homosexual males with HIV infection. There is a strong association between the appearance of these lesions and a history of receptive anal intercourse. the concomitant presence of anal human papillomavirus (HPV) is a risk for ASIL, which further increases when the CD4 lymphocyte count is lower. Progression of ASIL to HSIL can occur in 62% of HIV-infected males. Risks for progression include coinfection with multiple HPV types and a CD4 count < 200/microliter.

## Chorioretinitis

This is yet another complication that commonly develops in AIDS patients.

It is primarily caused by cytomegalovirus. It is usually bilateral, and frequently progress to blindness when retinae are extensively involved. Unfortunately, no treatment is available for it. However, patients receiving antiretroviral therapy resulting in a rise in CD4 lymphocyte counts may experience spontaneous healing of CMV retinitis lesions, even in the absence of anticytomegalovirus therapy. Such patients may also have atypical features of ocular CMV infection, including moderate to severe anterior chamber or vitreous inflammation. A so-called "immune recovery uveitis" may be observed in some patients undergoing successful highly active antiretroviral therapy (HAART), probably as a result of partial reconstitution of the immune system sufficient to allow an inflammatory reaction to develop against a previously subclinical CMV infection. Rare instances of chorioretinitis are caused by *Toxoplasma.*

## COMMON PATHOGENS

### Protozoa

***Pneumocystis carinii.*** It is the commonest (causing 60% opportunistic infections) organism infecting AIDS patients. Usually, it causes pneumonia, presenting with fever, chills, cough and dyspnoea. The duration of time between the onset of symptoms and documentation of *P. carinii* pneumonia, is characteristically longer in AIDS patients (median duration-28 days), when compared with the same in other immunocompromised hosts. Similarly, AIDS patients have lesser degree of tachypnoea and higher room air arterial oxygen concentrations than the latter group (Table 7.4).

**Table 7.4: The differences between *P. carinii* infections in AIDS and non-AIDS patients**

| Features | AIDS patients | Non-AIDS patients |
|---|---|---|
| 1. Duration of symptoms prior to diagnosis | Longer (median duration 28 days) | Shorter (median duration 5 days) |
| 2. Tachypoea | Less | Pronounced |
| 3. Arterial oxygen concentrations | Higher | Lower |
| 4. Duration of therapy | Longer | Relatively short |
| 5. Incidence of side-effects due to the therapy | Higher (rash: 30-80%, leucopenia uncorrected by leucovorin: 47-62%) | Lower |

*Pneumocystis carinii* in a ubiquitous extracellular protozoal which exists in the pulmonary alveoli as trophozoite or cyst forms. In the immunosuppressed hosts, it proliferates, thus, causing pneumonitis (PCP), revealed as diffuse alveolar infiltrates, or as interstitial densities in the skiagram of chest. In earlier stages, when chest X-rays are non-conclusive, gallium scan can be of immense value, and shows its greater uptake.

The gross pathology of the affected lung demonstrates that these tissues are heavy, consolidated diffuselly or in patches, and are cut with difficulty. Microscopic pathology reveals cysts of *P. carinii* within foamy eosinophilic exudates, distending alveoli and terminal bronchi. Occasional mononuclear and plasma cells can be seen within thickened alveolar septae. As PCP progresses, the lung texture becomes rubbery and the cut surfaces are often slimy, typical of diffuse alveolar damage (clinically defined as adult respiratory distress syndrome or "shock" lung). Severe infections poorly responsive to therapy may go on to produce diffuse alveolar damage that can organize to "honeycomb" lung with type II pneumonocyte hyperplasia and interstitial fibrosis.

Extrapulmonary spread of *P carinii* occurs in less than 5% of cases of AIDS. The most common site is hilar lymph nodes, spleen and liver. The microscopic appearance is often similar to that of the alveoli, but in widely disseminated cases, *P carinii* can produce numerous small 0.1 to 0.3 cm calcified granulomas that give the gross appearance of rough sandpaper to cut surfaces of parenchymal organs . A GMS stain reveals the organisms, even in densely calcified areas. Immunohistochemical staining of *P. carinii* in extrapulmonary sites is very useful.

Laboratory diagnosis can be done by demonstrating the organisms in frozen histopathologic sections of lung biopsy, or smears of pulmonary secretions (broncho-alveolar lavage specimens), using toluidine blue-O staining procedure. Transbronchial lung biopsy, although hazardous in a seriously ill patient, yet may be of immense value, for it may reveal other co-existing pulmonary pathogens. After its diagnosis is established with certainty a vigorous treatment is indicated, as outlined in chapter 11.

***Toxoplasma gondii:*** This protozoa has its natural habitat in animals. In AIDS patients, it can produce encephalitis, chorioretinitis, lymphadenopathy, or rarely disseminated toxoplasmosis. Toxoplasmosis is the most common etiology for focal brain lesions in AIDS, occurring in 30% to 40% of advanced AIDS patients. The prevalence of toxoplasmosis seen at autopsy has been decreasing with the use of prophylaxis, and now appears in less than 10% of cases. In most cases, toxoplasmosis in probably the result of reactivation of latent infection, since IgM antibodies are lacking. The central nervous system toxoplasmosis presents either as fulminant, subacute or chronic necrotizing encephalitis characterized by fever, seizures and focal neurological defects. Its differential diagnosis includes the abscesses produced by mycobacteria, cryptococcus, cytomegalovirus, and also lymphomas.

The demostration of *Toxoplasma* tachyzoites in the histologic sections of brain biopsy confirm its diagnosis, which, in addition, shows a well-demarcated necrotic area, with inflammatory cells and arteritis at the edges. The lumbar puncture is seldom fruitful, for it reveals only a mild, predominently mononuclear pleocytosis, normal or slightly low glucose and elevated protein levels. Computed tomographic scans of brain reveal single/multiple contrast-enhancing defects, either in homogeneous or ring pattern. Blood serology reveals a positive IgG-Sabin-Feldman dye test, but unlike non-AIDS toxoplasmosis patients, it seldom shows high titres.

The treatment of toxoplasmosis should be a prompt and prolonged course of pyrimethamine with sulfadiazine.

***Cryptosporidium:*** It is an enteric protozoan which may produce a persistent debilitating, profuse watery diarrhoea in AIDS patients. It is primarily a small bowel pathogen, and seldom escape to other organs. It usually causes wider-ranging symptoms of fever, nausea, vomiting, abdominal cramps and diarrhoea. The chronicity of symptoms may ultimately result in malabsorption, dehydration and death. The confirmation of the disease can be done by centrifugation of 0.5 g of stool specimen in sucrose solution, when the oocysts accumulate on the surface. They can be examined under microscope, after making a wet preparation of the surface film extracted with wire loop. The oocysts appear as brightly refractile, acid-fast, and contain characteristic dark granules. A small bowel biopsy reveals cryptosporidia arranged in rows, along the mucosal borders of blunted intestinal villi. Infrequently, cryptosporidia can also be identified in the gall bladder and tracheo-bronchial tree. However, they cannot be identified at autopsy, as autolysis separates them from the mucosal surfaces.

Spiramycin is the treatment of choice for cryptosporidiosis. It is given as one gram three times a day for one to 15 weeks. Nutritional supplementation, however, is of utmost importance.

***Other protozoa:*** In addition to *Pneumocystis carinii, Toxoplasma* and *Cryptosporidium,* other protozoa may also affect AIDS patients. They are *Giardia* and *Entamoeba,* chiefly manifesting as bowel symptoms. The bowel symptoms in AIDS patients may also be produced by bacteria such as *Campylobacter, Shigella* and *Salmonella,* which have to be kept as differential diagnosis.

## Fungi

***Candida albicans:*** Oral thrush is a common feature of most of the AIDS patients, which quite often extends to involve oesophagus. The patients who receive intravenous therapy, as well as severely cachectic and debilitated individuals may infrequently develop an invasive, widespread disease. The Centres for Disease Control qualifies the occurrence of candidial oesophagitis, or disseminated cadidiasis in a yough previously healthy, unmedicated patient, as a suspicion arouser of AIDS, as it is extremely rare in young, healthy men or women. The usual presentation of candidial oesophagitis is dysphagia, although it may sometimes be asymptomatic. A biopsy, however, has to be performed to differentiate it from oesophagitis due to *Herpes simplex* or *Cyto-megalovirus. Candidial* proctitis can be an occasional finding, when the patient presents with rectal pain, pruritus and purulent discharge.

The diagnosis of candidiasis should be established by the typical curdy-white appearance of surface of the lesions, whose removal reveals a raw, brigth-red area. There may be satellite pustules. the Gram-stained or wet-mounted scrapings reveal pseudohyphae and budding yeast cells. The biopsy specimen demonstrate typical 3-5 micron blastospores (budding yeast cells) and pseudohyphae, invading partially ulcerated epithelium.

***Crytococcus neoformans:*** This ubiquitous opportunistic fungus is a frequent cause of meningitis, encephalitis and disseminated infection in AIDS victims. Meningitis initially presents with a low grade fever and mild headache, followed by the development of nausea, vomiting and signs of meningeal involvemement. The analysis of the cerebrospinal fluid displays a mild pleocytosis, a high protein and a low glucose. India ink wet-mount preparation of the cerebrospinal fluid (CSF) reveals characteristic encapsulated, budding yeast forms. Serum and CSF cryptococcal antigen tests are almost always positive, as are the fungal cultures.

The biopsies of the infected tissues display intracellular and extracellular, 4-7 micron yeast forms with pale cell-wall. These cryptococcal yeast cells can be distinguished from those of *Blastomyces* and *Histoplasma*, by positive mucicarmine stains in the former. In addition, *C. neoformans* is surrounded by a characteristic carminophilic pink capsule, and possess narrow porebuds. The inflammation is conspicuously absent or minimal in AIDS patients. Computed tomography (CT) scans are usually of limited value. A disseminated infection has been demonstrated at autopsy, involving lungs, central nervous system, lymph nodes, adrenal glands, liver, spleen and bone marrow. A prompt and aggressive antifungal therapy is indicated after its diagnosis has been established.

***Histoplasma capsulatum:*** This fungus is found in soil contaminated by faeces of bats, chickens and starlings. Its infection is acquired in AIDS patients through inhalation of spores (microconidia). The organism gradually spreads from lungs to lymphnodes, liver, spleen, meninges, adrenal glands and bone-marrow through blood stream, culminating in disseminated histoplasmosis. These patients usually present with pyrexia of unknown origin (PUO), unexplained hepatosplenomegaly, abnormal liver function tests, chorioretinitis, meningitis, pancytopenia and lymph-node enlargement. The diagnosis of histoplasmosis can be established by the demonstration of typical oval, 2-4 micron, intracellular budding yeast cells within the reticuloendothelial system. These cells show a characteristic clear halo around them, caused by the retraction of the yeast protoplasm during fixation. The culture of the organisms is, however, difficult because of its fastidious nature.

***Coccidioides immitis:*** This soil fungus gains entry in the AIDS patients through inhalation of airborne arthrospores, commencing a primarily pulmonary infection. Further spread of the fungus occurs through haematogenous route to distant organs, Biopsy of the diseased tissue demonstrates 30-60 micron, thick-walled spherules, containing numerous endospores. In non-AIDS patients, there is an additional element of granulomatous caseation necrosis, which is conspicuously absent in AIDS patients, due to profound immunodepression.

***Aspergillus species:*** These ubiquitous molds may produce, in terminally ill AIDS patients, an invasive pulmonary infection. Due to their propensity to invade blood vessels, the infection soon disseminate to several distant organs, resulting in wedge-shaped lesions of several centimeters, with central necrosis. The frequency of aspergillosis, however, is no different than that seen in non-AIDS, immunocompromised hosts. The major clinical findings with pulmonary aspergillosis in AIDS are fever, cough, dyspnea in over half of cases. Other findings may include pleuritic chest pain, malaise, and weight loss. The two clinical patterns of pulmonary aspergillosis in AIDS are: (1) acute invasive pulmonary aspergillosis with prolonged cough and fever, and (2) obstructing-bronchial aspergillosis with dyspnea, cough (sometimes productive of bronchial casts containing the fungal hyphae), and chest pain. The diagnosis is confirmed by the demonstration of 3-4 micron, dichotomously branching septate hypae. They radiate peripherally from a central nidus, invading ruthlessly within the tissues, and occlude blood vessels through their passage in their walls.

***Nocardiosis:*** *Nocardia* can produce both localized and disseminated disease, usually late in the course of AIDS. The lung is the most common site for infection and *N asteroides* is the most frequent species isolated. There are no specific clinical features, though fever, productive cough, and weight loss are the most frequent findings. On chest radiograph, an alveolar pattern of pulmonary infiltrates is usual, with reticulonodular patterns seen in fewer patients. Gross pathologic features may include pneumonic consolidation, abscess formation, cavitation, and pleural effusions. Microscopically, *Nocardia* produces an acute inflammatory response in which the Gram positive filamentous organisms can be identified. The disease may remain localized or become disseminated to involve such sites as subcutaneous tissues, central nervous system, and kidney, with resultant high mortality rate. Early diagnosis from culture and treatment with sulfonamides or minocycline leads to better response and outcome.

## Viruses

***Cytomegalovirus:*** Nearly all patients of AIDS can be demonstrated to be infected with cytomegalovirus, as the virus can be cultured from either their throat, blood or urine. Nevertheless, it is difficult to ascribe a definitive disease process in all the AIDS patients from whom this virus is isolated. Several asymptomatic AIDS patients show a persistent viremia. However, it is believed to be a major cause of dysfunction in many organs of AIDS patients. In general population too, antibodies to *Cytomegalovirus* can be demonstrated in nearly 40-60 per cent, although it is rare to isolate the virus itself *in vitro*. In homosexual males, on the other hand, over 90 per cent show the antibody positivity, to which 30 per cent excrete the virus in their urine.

Fulminant *Cytomegalovirus* infections usually develop in late stages of full-blown AIDS, and carry an extremely poor prognosis. The commonest of cytomegalovirus diseases is pneumonitis, where lung biopsies reveal typical inclusion bodies that may be numerous in extensive and invariably fatal cases. Co-existence of cytomegalovirus infection with Kaposi's sarcoma or *P. carinii* infection is not unusual. It can also cause inflamation and ulceration of the gastro-intestinal mucosa, with occasional instances of perforation. Another serious complication, the chorioretinitis in AIDS is almost exclusively caused by this virus, displaying typical exudates and haemorrhages, with progressive visual loss Infection of the adrenal glands cause a massive, bilateral haemorrhagic necrosis, resulting in terminal hypotensive episodes in AIDS patients. The central nervous system affliction demonstrates initial subacute encephalitis, with progressive deterioration over a period of time. Microglial nodules can be seen in the grey matter. Other presentations of this viral infection may be fever, granulocytopenia, thrombocytopenic purpura, peripheral neuropathy and maculopapular rashes. Cytomegalovirus is known to be immunosuppressive, and thus might play a synergistic role in the generation of Kaposi's sarcoma and other malignancies. Autopsy of the patients dying of extensive cytomegalovirus infection demonstrates its inclusions in all tissues and organs of the body.

The diagnosis of pathological cytomegalovirus infection is usually established by the classical cytopathological changes observed in viral tissue cultures *in vitro,* and the demonstration of inclusion bodies at necropsy. The virus can be isolated from blood, urine and faeces, as well as from lungs, adrenal glands, eyes, central nervous system, gastrointestinal tract and male genitourinary system. Cytomegalovirus induces cellular gigantism (cytomegaly) with intranuclear and intracytoplasmic inclusions. Intranuclear inclusions are of a larger size and show eosinophilic staining in Haematoxylin-Eosin stains, and show a characteristic peripheral clear halo. They are amphophilic with PAS stain.

The management of cytomegalovirus infection has been a therapeutic enigma, as it has defied most of the antiviral drugs. Cyclovir derivatives, such as DHPG, however, hold some promise in the near future.

***Herpes simplex:*** Herpes simplex infection in AIDS may be primary or recurrent. The commonest presentation is a chronic mucocutaneous affliction or herpetic oesophagitis. The areas involved are the perianal region, followed by genital and oral mucocutaneous surfaces. These areas develop unusually extensive vesiculo-erosive lesions on an erythematous base. Proctitis caused by herpes simplex should, however, be differentiated from that caused by *Entamoeba histolytica, Chlamydia, Treponema pallida, Shigella, Campylobacter* and *Neisseria gonorrhoeae.*

The diagnosis of herpes simplex can be established by Tzanck test, and skin biopsy. Skin biopsy reveals an intraepidermal vesicle resulting from marked acantholysis and ballooning degeneration of epithelial cells. The balloon cells show enlarged nuclei containing eosinophilic inclusions surrounded by a clear halo (Cowdry type-A inclusion). Syncytial multinucleated giant cells may develop after coalition of infected cells.

***Herpes zoster:*** AIDS-patients, when develop recrudence of this virus, display unusually extensive herpes zoster, involving many dermatomes. Further, it shows a more prolonged course and delayed healing. The diagnosis of herpes zoster is fairly easy, and is based on characteristic grouped vesicles on an erythematous base, following dermatomal distribution. Tzanck test and histopathology shows results similar to those seen in herpes simplex.

***Molluscum contagiosum:*** AIDS patients infected with this DNA virus of the pox-virus group, show numerous 2-4 mm, domeshaped, umbilicated papules over the face and chest. Central cheeze core can be enucleated out with a needle. They may often attain a large size. The histopathology of these lesions is very salient.

***Condyloma acuminata:*** In AIDS patients, condyloma acuminata can be seen in perianal, genital or perioral location. They present as multiple soft, verrucous, cauliflower-like growths. Their diagnosis is fairly easy, and is based on characteristic clinical and histopathological features. The presence of vacuolated epithelial cells with hyperchromatic basophilic intranuclear inclusions, which may be shown to comprise of papillomavirus, are its diagnostic hallmarks.

***Polyoma virus:*** In immunocompromised hosts including AIDS patients, polyoma virus can cause progressive, multifocal leuko-encephalopathy. This starts with a slowly progressive dementia, indicating a diffuse but asymmetric disease. Computed tomography (CT) scans of the brain often reveal focal, hypodense white mater lesions, un-accompanied by contrast enhancement or mass effect. The histopathology demonstrates a granular, yellow softening of white mater on macroscopic examination, and patchy area of demyelination, necrosis and gliosis on microscopic examination.

***Epstein-Barr Virus:*** The role of this worlwide-existing herpesgroup DNA virus in AIDS and chronic lymphadenopathy syndrome is hitherto at best speculative. However, numerous AIDS and pre-AIDS patients have evidences favouring reactivated infection with Epstein-Barr virus, which is potentially immunosuppressive. It is implicated in polyclonal gammopathies of homosexual men, and also in Epstein-Barr virus-associated lymphomas of AIDS. Seroepidemiologic evidence suggests that Epstein-Barr virus infections are fairly common in young children. Clinical infections can be diagnosed by determination of serologic titres, detection of viral antigens, and by direct viral isolation. Polyclonal activation of B-cells, and transformation of cultured lymphocytes into permanent cell-lines suggests an *in vitro* infection of human lymphocytes by this virus.

***Hepatitis-B virus:*** The male homosexuals as well as intracvenous drug injectors render themselves at-risk for introducing hepatitis-B infection in their body. The mode of transmission of this agent is through various means to transfer of infected body secretion, akin to the transmission of AIDS. However, the concurrent occurrence of hepatitis-B infection in AIDS patients has hardly any remarkable clinico-epidemiological or therapeutic significance for the reason that (i) AIDS patients lack effector cells responsible for the damaging sequelae of hepatitis-B infection, and thus do not exhibit either chronic-persistent or chronic-active hepatitis, or cirrhosis, and (ii) the precautions to be taken in management and prevention of hepatitis-B patients are equally or even more seriously necessary in AIDS patients.

## Bacteria

***Mycobacterium avium-intercellulare:*** This ubiquitous, atypical acid-fast mycobacteria can be differentiated from *Mycobacterium tuberculosis* by its cultural characteristics including its slow growing, non-photochromogenic character. It was exceptional to observe infections caused by this mycobacteria prior to the 'era' of AIDS. Its infections were, however, sporadically seen in patients with ectatic lung diseases causing chronic cavitary fibronodular pulmonary affection. In contrast, it is fairly common (20 per cent of the opportunistic infections) in AIDS patients, that too in a disseminated form. It usually presents with pyrexia, anorexia, weight loss and debilitation. Other concurrent infections, nevertheless, divert the attention of the treating physician, and thus it may escape recognition and therapy. But once diagnosed, its specific treatment may cause rapid improvement of the general health. Occasionally, *M. avium-intercellulare* may cause pneumonitis, and sometimes chronic diarrhoes with Whipple's-like syndrome.

The diagnosis of this atypical mycobacteria is established by culture of the blood, urine, bone marrow, lymphnode or other appropriate biopsy tissue. Positive culture from sputum alone is not conclusive, as it can be a saprophyte in the bronchial tree. The culture grows fairly rapid (2-3 weeks, especially blood and bone marrow cultures), if lysis-centrifugation or radiometric culture system is employed. The microscopy of infected tissues characteristically demonstrates sheets of foamy histiocytes with minimal inflammatory infiltrate, conspicuous by the absense of granulomas so characteristic of other mycobacterial infections. Acid-fast stain reveals a large number of mycobacteria in the cytoplasm of these histiocytes.

***Mycobaterium tuberculosis:*** Developing countries still have sufficient quantum of tuberculous infections. Thus, if the *Mycobaterium tuberculosis* infection supervenes in AIDS patient, the underlying immunodeficiency might be overlooked in the developing countries. It, thus, warrants a high degree of suspicion, when tuberculosis develops in a hitherto healthy young adult. Studies conducted at AIDS Research and Control (ARCON) Centre at Sir J.J. Hospital, Mumbai, show that the annual incidence of tuberculosis in an HIV-infected prevalent cohort studied longitudinally is 8.5/100 person years; a lifetime risk of developing tuberculosis (TB) is approximately 60 per cent and postmortem examinations of established tuberculosis as the predominant cause of death in 73.9% cases of AIDS. Tuberculous infection, however, has not frequently been recognised in AIDS patients of the United States. Nevertheless, this infection is commonly found in AIDS patients of Haiti origin. The disseminated/ extrapulmonary tuberculosis may manifest before other clinical manifestations of AIDS. The microscopic appearance of *M. tuberculosis* closely mimic *M. avium intracellular* and thus both cannot be easily distinguished.

HIV fuels the TB epidemic. The rate of progression to active TB is 10 to 30 times higher among individuals infected by both TB and HIV than among those infected only with TB. This is because people with HIV infection have suppressed immunity and hence chances of reactivation of dormant TB bacilli is many fold higher in them, Due to low immunity, natural infection may rapidly lead to TB disease. HIV infection may also contribute to an increase in drug resistance. Increased TB cases in HIV-infected people pose risk of TB transmission to others in the general community.

As the HIV infection progresses, the CD4 lymphocytes decline in number and function. Therefore, the immune system is less able to prevent the growth and spread of the TB bacilli. As a result, disseminated and extra-pulmonary TB disease is more commonly seen in the later stages. Studies have shown that pulmonary involvement occurs in 70-90 percent of all HIV/AIDS patients with TB.

Recognizing the serious threat posed by HIV-TB co-infection, the Government of India has emphasized the need for strengthening collaboration between TB and AIDS control programs for better management of HIV-infected patients with TB. Efforts are being made to establish Voluntary Counselling & Testing for HIV, diagnosis for TB and Direct Observed Treatment-short course for TB to make such services available to the needy patients.

Laboratory diagnosis of pulmonary tuberculosis in HIV-infected persons can be most easily made with sputum samples and detection of acid-fast bacilli under fluorescence microscopy with the auramine stain. Most such infections can be detected with a single specimen. The chemotherapy of tuberculosis is by combined antitubercular drugs regimen for 9 to 18 months' duration. The relapses, however, may be anticipated. Cases of multidrug resistant tuberculosis are also reported and have to be kept in mind in case of a relapse. Levels of drug resistance are rising globally. India has been declared as a "hot spot" for multidrug resistant tuberculosis (MDR-TB). HIV-infected patients are at an increased risk of acquiring drug resistant TB due to low level of CMI. Studies among the dually infected patients conducted at ARCON, Mumbai, in collaboration with Foundation for Medical Research, reveal that a high level (72%) of patients were resistant to 4 to 5 second line anti-tuberculosis drugs. Drug resistance to individual drug was high ranging from 62 to 100 per cent. Another study conducted at Sir J.J. Hospital on MDR-TB showed drug resistance among 35% of strains tested.

***Other Bacteria:*** *Legionella,* Gram positive cocci, *Salmonella,* and *Shigella* have also been seen to infect AIDS patients with increased frequency. *Salmonella* species (not *typhi*) can occur in persons at risk for HIV infection, but most often after clinical AIDS is apparent. Gastrointestinal *Salmonella* infections with high fever have a propensity to result in septicemia and to relapse, particularly when CD4 lymphocyte counts are low. Recurrent *Salmonella* infection is a criterion for diagnosis of AIDS in adults and children.

*Shigella* infections tend to occur early with HIV infection, and half may be accompanied with bacteremia. *Campylobacter jejuni* can produce a proctocolitis, and patients often do not have fever. *Clostridium dificile* infection may develop in AIDS patients treated with broad spectrum antibiotics, may produce pseudomembranous colitis, and may not respond promptly to therapy. The bacteria affecting AIDS patients may, however, differ from one geographic area to other, depending upon their prevalence. They often produce unusual pattern of infections in these patients.

***Genital Ulcer Disease vs. HIV infection:*** All major genital disease viz syphilis, genital herpes and chancroid have been shown to be associated with an increased risk of transmitting HIV infection, which may be upto 3 to 5 times. Sexually transmitted infections (STIs) may enhance both the acquisition as well as transmission of HIV. This relationship is especially true of STIs causing genital ulcers. STIs in HIV-seropositive persons may differ qualitatively or quantitatively, or both, in both clinical and laboratory parameters from sexually transmitted diseases (STDs) in immuncompetent persons. Such measures as education, which may lead to early recognition of the signs and symptoms of STIs, have the potential to positively affect the HIV epidemic. Therefore enhanced efforts should be devoted to the prevention and treatment of STIs.

Precise data about the prevalence of STIs in India is not available. However, from the limited number of studies conducted among the 'High Risk Population' or 'Hospital Based Studies' prevalence rate of STIs in India has been quoted to be about five percent. Now, NACO has planned to ascertain the prevalence of STIs and also health seeking behaviour of persons suffering from this group of diseases by undertaking a country wide Community Based STI Prevalence Survey. STD Control Programme is based on early diagnosis and prompt treatment of STIs and relies on the health seeking behaviour of individuals with STD. It is directly related to the stigma attached to the disease, because of which, individuals with STI desire anonymity. As a result, they seek alternate source of medical aid including self-medication and only a small proportion report to public sector medical set up. Because of this attitude and behaviour of those suffering from STIs, majority who should have been adequately treated and rendered non-infectious escape treatment and continue transmitting infection to their multiple sex partners. Under the STD Control Programme the government has established STD Clinic in each District Hospital, all over the country. The STI drugs are provided free of cost by Govt of India and adequate confidentiality is ensured for those attending these clinics. STDs facilitate the HIV transmission either by increasing HIV susceptibility or HIV infectiousness or both. HIV infection also alters the natural history, manifestations and treatment of different STDs. By treating all STDs at the earliest, HIV transmission can be prevented by 40 to 50 per cent, especially in early epidemic phase.

***In substance:*** The majority of individuals do not experience signs and symptom at the time of primary infection. However, some may develop fever, rigors, athralgias, diarrhoea, and aseptic meningitis 3 to 6 weeks after infection. These constitutional symptoms may last for 2 to 3 weeks and then resolve spontaneously.

The acute illness of primary infection is followed by a period of asymptomatic infection. Eight to ten years may elapse before the development of full-blown AIDS. However, 80 to 90 per cent of the infected patients will reveal immunologic deterioration within 3 years of infection, though the clinical symptoms may be lacking. Approximately 75 per cent of infected individuals develop some symptoms within the first 7 years. Thus, the acquired immunodeficiency patients make themselves prone to get infected with various micro-organisms-virus, bacteria, fungi and protozoa-due to their aberrant cellular immune function, as they are unable to resist their invasion. The patient may get afflicted by several infections at a time, and may also have coexistent malignancy, making the net clinical scenario more bizarre and complicated. Only keeping such an intriguing possibility in mind will assist in complete diagnosis, and thus prompt eradication of such infections in their unimaginable permutations and combinations.

# 8

# Cancers
# The Added Agony

The immunodeficiency acquired by the invasion of HIV-1 virus, seriously impair the immune surveillance of these patients, thus, facilitating the prohibited clones of abnormal cells to reproduce at a prolific rate. This results in the development of bizarre malignancies. Such malignancies, otherwise, have a very low incidence in the general population.

## KAPOSI'S SARCOMA

Ever since its inception in the year 1872 by an Hungarian Dermatologist Moriz Kaposi, Kaposi's sarcoma has remained an unusual and rare tumour. Its recent resurgence, as an epidemic of a disseminated and fulminant form occurring in young homosexual men, was one major factor that led to the discovery of AIDS. This outbreak was too surprising, as it happened in large urban centres of the United States. This was then designated as epidemic Kaposi's sarcoma.

### Incidence

The AIDS-related Kaposi's sarcoma has been seen in individuals as young as 19 years, and as old as 64 years, with a mean age-of-onset of 37.7 years. Nearly 48 per cent of AIDS-afflicted homosexual males develop this malignancy, while about 4% and 12% of heterosexual intravenous drug abusers and Haitians respectively develop it. In paediatric age group, its incidence is roughly 5 per cent.

The adult patients have been found to be sexually promiscuous, and have history of multiple sexually-transmitted diseases in the past. They may also have a history of sexual practices involving exposure to faecal matter, such as anal lingus, anal intercourse and fist fornication. It appears that the exposure of rectal mucosa to semen during anogenital intercourse increases the risk of development of epidemic Kaposi's sarcoma.

## Clinical Features

The epidemic Kaposi's sarcoma has to be differentiated from the three other varieties (Table 8.1). There are wide variations in their age of onset, clinical features, course and response to therapy, and thus the diagnosis may not be difficult. Kaposi's sarcoma is defined as a multi-focal, factor VIII producing vascular tumour of the integument, mucous membranes, lymphnodes and the internal viscera. A role of the immune response genes is suggested in the pathogenesis of this neoplasm, as an increased incidence of HLA-DRS is seen in these patients. Epidemic (AIDS-related) Kaposi's sarcoma displays certain morphologic peculiarities. Systemic manifestation such as pyrexia of unknown origin, weight loss, diarrhoea, malaise, and fatigue may precede or occur at its onset. Certain skin lesions viz. impetigo, vague psoriasiform or pruritic, eczematous skin eruptions, superficial fungal infections of skin and nails, and oral/ oesophageal candidiasis may herald its onset. Other viral infections may also occur concomitantly.

The skin tumours vary from pink to deep-purple papules and nodules, with an areola of brown pigmentation. In addition, they may develop subcutaneous ecchymoses (in the absence of thrombocytopenia or history of trauma). The early flat lesions may actually be mistaken for pityriasis rosea, purpura, pigmented naevi, Schamberg's disease, early melanoma, secondary syphilis, or flat haemangiomas. In the advancing phase, in addition to papules and nodules, macules, patches and plaques can also develop. Not infrequently, the lesions in the dependent areas may discharge serosanguinous fluid, and get infected. They, otherwise, are asymptomatic. The initial favoured sites are ankles and soles of the feet, but later the lesions may disseminate to any area of the body. As the lesions become numerous, they seem to become bilateral and symmetrical, along the lines of skin cleavage. The richly vascular impression of these lesions seems deceptive, as they bleed only rarely. A fungation with ulceration may be expected in older lesions. Similar lesions occur in the oral mucosa, lymphnodes and internal viscera of the body, particularly gastrointestinal tract, lungs and liver. Oral lesions are common on the hard and soft palate, gingival and buccal mucosa, tonsils and pharynx.

**Table 8.1: The differentiation of epidemic Kaposi's sarcoma with other variants**

| Features | Epidemic (AIDS) | Classic | African | Renal Transplant |
|---|---|---|---|---|
| Age-group | Young adults primarily homosexuals | 50-80 years | Young adults (25-40 years) as well as children (2-13 years) | Immunosuppressed subjects of any age. |
| Geographic area | Any area | Jewish & Italian | Central Africa | Jewish & Mediterranean |
| Sex ratio (male:female) | Mainly Males | 10-15:1 | 13:1 in adults; 3:1 in children | 2-3:1 |
| Morphologic peculiarities | Disseminated, with involvement of lymph nodes and viscera | Confined to lower limbs with venous stasis; later wide-spread cutaneous & systemic lesions | Adults: Localized nodular lesions; children: Generalised lesions | May be localized to skin or have widespread systemic disease. |
| Course | Fulminant (20% survival after 2 years) | Indolent (Survival for 10-15 years) | Adults: indolent<br>Children: rapidly fatal | May be indolent or rapidly progressive |
| Treatment | Systemic Chemotherapy | Irradiation, surgical excision, or electro-cauterization | Adults: Chemotherapy; Children: rapidly fatal even with combination chemotherapy | Radiotherapy |
| Prognosis | Discouraging | Relatively better | Adults: good<br>Children: very poor | Guarded |

## Histopathology

The histopathological features of epidemic Kaposi's sarcoma are no different than those of the 3 other forms. Well-developed lesions show a very few thin, endothelium-lined vascular slits. surrounded and compressed by dense, interweaving bundles or fascicles of spindle-shaped cells. The developing lesions, however, show numerous irregular vascular slits. Red blood cells can be seen in them. In addition, there is a dense mononuclear inflammatory cell infiltrate, composed primarily of plasma cells and lymphocytes, present throughout the dermis. Indirect immunoperoxidase technique reveals the presence of Factor VIII in the spindle-shaped cells as well as the endothelial cells.

## Staging

Kaposi's sarcoma (KS) has been divided into 4 stages. Stage I represents a cutaneous, locally indolent classic Kaposi's sarcoma, common in elderly males of Mediterranean or East European origin. Stage II represents African Kaposi's sarcoma in its locally malignant forms. Stage III and IV include the disseminated and systemic Kaposi's sarcoma, observed in AIDS as well as the African children. Subdivisions A and B are designated to each stage, where A signify no systemic signs, while B point to systemic signs including over 10% weight loss, and greater than 100°F fever of unknown origin for over 2 weeks. On this scale, the percentage and survival rate of AIDS-related Kaposi's sarcoma can be roughly expected as shown in Table 8.2.

**Table 8.2: Stage-wise incidence and prognosis of epidemic Kaposi's sarcoma**

| State | Incidence (%) | Survival rate at 2 years (%) |
|---|---|---|
| I | 10-15 | 100 |
| II | 10-30 | 90 |
| III-A | 20-25 | 60 |
| III-B | 10-12 | 16 |
| IV-A | 20-25 | 60 |
| IV-B | 10-12 | 16 |

Prognosis is variable in different stages, signifying that the extent of the disease, the presence/absence of systemic symptoms, and the presence of opportunistic infections have a major impact on its prognosis. The

# 9

# AIDS-Related Complex (ARC) – An Early Clue

The AIDS-related complex (ARC) can be regarded as a milder form of AIDS, reflecting either a distinct syndrome of unexplained lymphadenopathy, fatigue, fever and weight loss, or idiopathic thromobocytopenic purpura. A patient should be designated as ARC if he fulfils its criteria of two clinical features with two AIDS-specific laboratory abnormalities (Table 9.1). The so called lymphadenopathy syndrome (LAS) thus falls under this category. The term LAS is labelled to patients having lymphadenopathy (nodes of diameter one cm or more) affecting 2 or more extrainguinal, non-contiguous sites, and present for 3 months or more, and for which no known cause can be ascribed. This is commonly seen in intravenous drug abusers, Haitians, haemophiliacs, prisoners, female partners of men with AIDS, and their infants. The chief complaints of LAS patients are the enlargement of lymph nodes, associated with chronic fatigue and flu-like illness. Such a situation may, however, not be infrequent in the developing countries, including India. Nevertheless, all the known causes of chronic lymph node enlargement should be excluded before designating it as a manifestation of AIDS. Most of these patients characteristically give history of (a) past sexual activities with multiple partners, (b) recurrent sexually-transmitted diseases, and/or (c) frequent use of recreational drugs.

The symptoms, in order of frequency, include fatigue, night sweats, flu-like illness, fever and weight loss. Splenomegaly may be apparent in one third of these patients. Other conditions commonly seen in these patients include recurrent minor bacterial and fungal infections, herpes simplex, seborrhoeic dermatitis, genital warts and episodes of herpes zoster. Neuropsychiatric symptoms are an additional pointer, but occur only in a minority. They are anxiety, depression, severe headaches and unexplained inflammatory polyneuropathy.

**Table 9.1: AIDS-related complex (ARC)**

| | Clinical Features | Laboratory Abnormalities |
|---|---|---|
| 1. | Fever over 100°F for 3 months | Helper-T-cells below 400/$mm^3$ |
| 2. | Over 10% weight loss (15 pounds or more) | Helper: Suppressor ratio less than 1. |
| 3. | Lymphadenopathy of over 3 months | Leukopenia, thrombocytopenia, anaemia |
| 4. | Diarrhoea | Elevated serum globulins |
| 5. | Fatigue | Depressed blastogenesis |
| 6. | Night sweats | Anergy to skin tests |

Criteria of Diagnosis: two clinical features + two laboratory abnormalities

The affected lymph nodes are enlarged, firm/soft, discrete, mobile and non-tender. The affliction of cervical, axillary and inguinal lymph nodes is usually a common denominator. On an average, however, 10 nodal sites are affected. Retroperitoneal lymphnodes involvement can be demonstrated in abdominal CT scans, although mediastinal adenopathy may not be discernible.

## LABORATORY INVESTIGATIONS

The laboratory abnormalities are generally unremarkable. Haematologic abnormalities of various grades, howeyer, may be discovered, with mild elevation of liver enzymes. A polyclonal increase in gammaglobulin levels (lgG & lgA) may be a constant finding. A cutaneous anergy to various recall skin test antigens can also be demonstrated, as is the lowered $CD_4$: $CD_8$ lympocyte phenotype ratio. A diminished *in vitro* lymphocyte responses to T-cell and B-cell mitogens are also a feature of ARC.

The virologic and serologic studies reveal a universal exposure to cytomegalovirus and Epstein-Barr virus, with grossly raised lgG levels. The antibodies to HIV-1 can be demonstrated in all the patients with ARC, relating it strongly to AIDS. The culture of the lymphnode materials for bacteria or fungi, to rule out infectious causes of lymphadenopathy, are uniformly negative.

The CD4+ T-lymphocyte count is generally regarded as the best market for the progression of HIV-related disease. As the CD4+ T-cell count declines, the risk for developing a broad spectrum of illnesses, including those meeting the AIDS-defining criteria, increases. Monitoring CD4+ T-cell counts is part of the recommended standard of care for persons with HIV infection, and CD4+ T-cell counts are used to guide clinical decisions regarding the use of antiretroviral therapy and prophylaxis against *Pneumocystis carinii.* Estimates of the number of persons with CD4+ T-cell counts < 200 cells/μL but without AIDS are therefore needed for public health planning.

## HISTOPATHOLOGY

The histopathological examination of the affected lymph nodes reveal a marked follicular hyperplasia with large cleaved and non-cleaved lymphocytes, macrophages and immunoblasts. Other patterns of histopathological changes can also be encountered in the lymph nodes of LAS patients, which some pathologists regard only as evolutionary changes developing over a period of time. The presence of follicular involution (or folliculysis) with the depletion of lymphocytes warrant the progression of the disease to full-blown AIDS, and may also herald the development of B-cell lymphomas.

## IMMUNOPATHOGENESIS

A battery of complicated immunological investigations performed on the patients with AIDS-related complex reveal that it can conveniently be placed at the junction of immunocompetency merging slowly into the spectrum of AIDS, leading to severe immunodeficiency. The $CD_4$; $CD_8$ lymphocyte ratio in LAS range from 0.4:1 to 1.1:1, attributable primarily to the depletion of $CD_4$ cells, with some increase of $CD_8$ cells. Further, T-cell responses to mitogens and antigens *in vitro* are low. The pathogenesis of affliction of $CD_4$ lymphocyte sub-population is similar to that occurs in AIDS.

## DIFFERENTIAL DIAGNOSIS

Lymphadenopathy syndrome has to be distinguished from other viral illnesses such as Epstein-Barr virus, cytomegalovirus and cat-scratch fever, which may show similar characteristics. Further, a confusing picture may also arise in tuberculosis, toxoplasmosis, crytococcosis, typhoid and syphilis, all of which produce a generalised lymphadenopathy.

## FOLLOW UP

All suspected patients of ARC should compulsorily be followed up for a period of 1 to 3 years for the development of overt symptoms of AIDS. It is believed that about 7 to 17 per cent of ARC patient will land up in AIDS in about 2 years, the conversion is usually ushered in by the onset of a wasting syndrome, characterised by regression of lymphadenopathy, extreme fatigue, sweating, fever and weight loss.

# 10

# Diagnostic Approach

The diagnosis of AIDS should only be established after eliciting unequivocal signs, symptoms, and positive diagnostic tests. It should be strongly stressed that in no case any patient should be labelled as AIDS merely on either suspicion, circumstantial evidence or equivocal laboratory investigations. Further, the syndrome of persistent generalised lymphadenopathy (PGL) is regarded as an early manifestation of AIDS, as about one-third to one-half of AIDS patients reveal an antecedent lymphadenopathy syndrome (LAS) for 6-18 months prior to the appearance of full-blown picture of AIDS. This has also been designated as AIDS-related complex (ARC). The diagnosis of AIDS and ARC is thus made on history, clinical assessment and laboratory investigations.

## HISTORY

History can lucidly elicit that the suspected patient belongs to a known high-risk group, viz. homosexual male, parentral drug abuser, haemophiliac, recipient of repeated blood/blood products transfusion, Haitian, female partner of AIDS-patients and their offsprings. It also clarifies that this patient was a previously healthy young man or woman, without any known cause of congenital or acquired immunodeficiency i.e. receiving immunosuppressive agents etc. An exposure to a known AIDS-patient may also be elicitable in the history.

## CLINICAL EXAMINATION

Clinical assessment may often baffle the treating physician, for the patient displays unusually extensive infections, which respond far from satisfactory to the usual chemotherapeutic agents, while the patient keeps on deteriorating, suggesting an utter immune system failure of his body. Moreover, they are caused by microbes which normally do not prefer human body, or attack only a severely immunocompromised host. Alternatively, he may present with malignancies that are only exceptional to his age and are developing at a fairly rapid rate, at multiple sites. An alert physician can suspect the syndrome, even when patient presents in the prodromal stages, manifesting with recurrent herpes/candidiasis. Or, the patient may reveal lymph node enlargement, which persist despite treatment, and for which no known cause can be incriminated. (Table 10.1) The detailed clinical features of AIDS and ARC are discussed in the chapter 4,5 and 9. They should be taken cogniscence of in the clinical examination in details, for reaching a conclusive diagnosis.

**Table 10.1: Suggestive clinical findings of HIV infection**

a. Fever of over one month's duration
b. Weight loss of more than 10%
c. Diarrhoea of more than one month's duration
d. Mucocutaneous manifestations
e. Generalised lymphadenopathy (extra-inguinal)
f. Infections, severe or recurrent, unusual
g. Unexplained neurological manifestations e.g. seizures, motor or sensory deficits, dementia and progressive headache
h. Chronic cough of more than one month's duration or unexplained respiratory distress
i. Cytomegalovirus retinitis
j. Extrapulmonary or disseminated and extensive pulmonary tuberculosis
k. Recurrent pneumonia
l. Invasive cervical carcinoma.

Apart from CDC revised classification (Chapter 1), Walter Reed's (WR) classification is also *in vogue.* The patient is thoroughly examined for the clinical manifestations of HIV disease, screened for antibodies to HIV using ELISA, the positive results of which are then confirmed by Western blot, a T-helper cell count is obtained, and also anergy screening is done by skin testing with mumps, tetanus, trichophyton, and monilial antigens. (Table 10.2)

**Table 10.2: Walter Reed's Classification**

| | |
|---|---|
| WR0: | antibody negative patient with sexual contact with patient with HIV infection. |
| WR1: | positive culture for, or 2 positive Western blots to HIV. |
| WR2: | 2 positive Western blots and chronic lymphadenopathy |
| WR3: | 2 positive Western blots and persistent T-helper cell depletion. |
| WR3: | 2 positive Western blots, persistent T-helper cell depletion and partial defects in delayed hypersensitivity (DH). |
| WR5: | 2 positive Western blots, T-helper cell depletion, and either a clinical thrush or persistent energy. |
| WR6: | 2 positive Western blots and an opportunistic infection. |

The world Health Organization has laid criteria for the case definition of clinical AIDS. An AIDS-positive individual has been identified as meeting the two criteria A and B below:

A. Positive test for HIV infection by two tests based on preferably two different antigens.

B. Any one of the following criteria:

1. (a) Weight loss of 10% body weight or cachexia, not known to be due to a condition unrelated to HIV infection

   (b) Chronic diarrhoea of one month's duration, intermittent or constant
2. Disseminated, miliary or extrapulmonary tuberculosis
3. Candidiasis of the oesophagus; diagnosable as dysphagia, odynophagia and oral candidiasis
4. Neurological impairment restricting daily activities, not known to be due to a condition unrelated to HIV (e.g. trauma)
5. Kaposi's sarcoma

## LABORATORY INVESTIGATIONS

The diagnosis of HIV infection is accomplished by performing a battery of diagnostic tests. Diagnostic tests for human immunodeficiency virus (HIV) infection use four approaches: identification of antibodies to viral proteins, detection of viral antigens, detection of viral nucleic acids and culturing the virus. (Table 10.3).

The HIV testing can be performed in any patient whc requests it or where we suspect that there are indication for testing it (Table 10.4).

**Table 10.3: Laboratory tests for diagnosing HIV infection**

| Test | Characteristics |
|---|---|
| 1. ELISA | Primary screening tool for diagnosis |
| 2. Western Blot | Confirmatory test when ELISA is positive |
| 3. HIV p24 antigen | Poor sensitivity; previously used to help establish diagnosis in persons with negative serologic tests, and to provide prognostic data in persons with established HIV infection |
| 4. Qualitative assay (DNA PCR) | For early diagnosis; diagnosing vertically transmitted HIV infection in neonates at risk; as a confirmatory assay to supplement serologic diagnosis; research purposes |
| 5. Quantitative assays (RT PCR) | Measuring viral load |
| 6. HIV culture | Highly specific but relatively insensitive for diagnosis; difficult; research purposes |

**Table 10.4: Indications for HIV antibody screening**

**Behaviours associated with increased risk**

- People with multiple sexual partners
- People with recent or prior sexually transmitted infections
- Commercial sex workers and their partners
- Men who have sex with men
- Travellers who visited areas of increased prevalence and were sexually active
- Injection drug users
- Sexual partners of at-risk persons
- Recipients of blood products prior to HIV screening

**Routine screening recommended to discover low risk persons with unanticipated infection**

- Pregnant women
- Donors of blood products, semen, ova or organs
- Patients hospitalized in an area with more than 1/1000 HIV prevalence

*(Contd.)*

*(Table 10.4 Contd.)*

| **Clinical conditions associated with increased risk behaviour or occult immunocompromise** |
|---|
| • Sexually transmitted infection |
| • Thrush or chronic/recurrent vulvovaginal candidiasis |
| • Generalized lymphadenopathy |
| • Recurrent herpes simplex or herpes zoster |
| • Tuberculosis |
| • Constitutional symptoms such as pyrexia of unknown origin and unexplained weight loss |
| • Chronic diarrhoea or wasting |
| • Encephalopathy |
| • Anaemia, leukopenia or thrombocytopenia |
| • Opportunistic infections |

## Demonstration of antibodies to HIV-1

It is based on the fact that both humoral and cell-mediated immunity respond to counter any viral infection, with the formation of antibodies against viral antigens. Antibodies may form against many antigenic components. However, their amount varies with the quantum of antigenic components. Thus, the maximum antibody response is seen to that protein fraction which is abundant. The central core of the virion chiefly contain the antigenic components, constituted by viral RNA reverse transcriptase and several smaller nucleic-acid-binding proteins. There are 3 group-specific antigens of HIV-1, of which the major core antigen $P^{24}$ (protein of molecular weight 24,000 daltons) forms an integral part. The other 2 are derived from the envelop, constituted by the major surface glycoproteins linked non-covalently to the transmembrane protein. The quantitation of antibody response can be measured by various tests:

**(i) Enzyme-linked immunosorbence assay (ELISA) tests:** This sensitive test is useful in screening large number of individuals for HIV infection. More than 95 per cent of HIV infected persons will be identified as positive by ELISA within 3 months of infection. Its major disadvantage is a relatively high incidence of false positive reactions. The rate of false positive reactions with first generation ELISA, which employs lysates from the HIV infected cells as a source of antigen, has been reduced with second generation ELISA, that utilizes recombinant DNA protein as a source of antigen. All positive ELISA tests should be repeated and if the repeat test is also positive, it should by confirmed by a more specific test for the antibody.

Elisa test has the advantage that it measures antibodies to all viral proteins. It employs the absorption of the components of this virion or the detergent-disrupted virus to the wells in plastic dishes. Then, these are reacted with an unknown human serum. Subsequently, an antihuman globulin serum with attached enzyme is added. In the last step, a calorimetric agent is added to it. If human serum had got bound to the virus, then the reagent also binds to it, causing the development of colour, and thus a positive test. It is relatively simple test, and also a sensitive one. A rapid calorimetric test is automated, which can be performed in any volume, and is the method of choice for testing the donated blood.

**(ii) Western electroblot test:** The Western Blot test detected antibodies to individual HIV antigens that are separated into distinct bands by electrophoresis. The presence of any two to the p24, gp41 and gp 120/gp 160 bands is considered a positive result. The absence of all bands is a negative test. An indeterminate test has a single band or other bands not included in the definition of a positive test. Indeterminate tests may represent nonspecific antibody reactions, may result from testing individuals with recently acquired HIV-1 infection, or may result from infection with HIV-2. A positive ELISA combined with an unambiguously positive Western Blot is conclusive evidence for HIV infection. Conversely, an unambiguously negative Western Blot combined with a positive screening assay suggests that the ELISA result was falsely positive.

Here, the viral proteins are separated by electrophoresis. They are subsequently reacted with the human sera, causing the formation of antigen-antibody complexes. This is then transferred to a membrane, where the complex is identified by using a radioactively-labelled protein having a high degree of affinity for this complex, such as *Staphylococcus*-A proteins. The major reactivity detected, is seen to be directed against the viral envelop glycoprotein of molecular weight 41,000 (gp 41). The $P^{24}$, however, is not recognised so well by this test. (Table 10.5)

**(iii) Radioimmune assays:** The radioimmune assays of HIV-1 have been found to be both sensitive and specific. In addition, these tests are fairly rapid. However, this test measures antibody to only a single viral protein, thus picking only one-half of AIDS and three-quarter of ARC/LAS patients. This makes the test less sensitive than Western blot or ELISA test. This test employs a purified radiolabelled viral protein, usually core $p^{24}$. An antibody is developed against this component in an animal species. The human antibody then competes for the labelled reaction, thus measuring the response to a single viral protein.

**Table 10.5: Evolution of markers for HIV infection**

| | Stage of Infection | p24 antigen | anti-HIV | Western blot pattern |
|---|---|---|---|---|
| 1. | Soon after infection | – → + | – | – |
| 2. | Acute illness | + → – | ± → + | Restricted, often p24 and/or gp 120 |
| 3. | Asymptomatic carrier | – | + | Full pattern |
| 4. | Symptomatic carrier | + | + | Loss of anti p24 |
| 5. | AIDS | + | + | Absence of anti-p24 |

**(iv) Immunofluorescence Test:** It was the first definitive test to tie the reactivity of human serum to HIV infected cells. The presently used modifications of this test are highly sensitive. In this test, a human target cell is infected with live or fixed virus. It is then reacted with human serum. A fluorescein-labelled anti-human globulin can demonstrate the binding as a 'sandwich'. The antigens on the cell membrane of live cells are best detected by this test.

**(v) Polymerase chain reaction (PCR) assays:** The PCR technique is used to assay for both HIV RNA and HIV DNA. The only test to diagnose HIV infection in the window period (i.e. when antibodies to HIV have not yet developed and ELISA is negative) is the HIV DNA PCR. However, even this test may be negative during the first week after viral entry.

The HIV RNA PCR test can measure the amount of HIV RNA in the blood (also referred to as the "viral load"). The viral load indicates the rate of disease progression, with higher viral loads predictive of faster disease progression. HIV RNA PCR is also used to assess the response to anti-HIV therapy. The viral load may also be measured using another technique known as the branched DNA (bDNA) technique.

## Isolation of HIV-1

This is the most specific marker of the diagnosis of AIDS. It can be recovered from over 85 per cent of early AIDS and 30 per cent of fulminant AIDS patients. A low frequency of isolation of live virus in late stages of AIDS is chiefly due to the fact that the $OKT_4^+$ cells population, that harbour it, is profoundly diminished.

Viral culture is a highly specific but relatively insensitive means of diagnosing HIV infection. Success rates are highly variable due to varying degrees of viremia at different stages of HIV infection and the difficulties of proper collection and transport of the blood before culture.

In general, AIDS patients are uniformly positive for the antibodies to HIV-1. However, their titres fall significantly in terminal AIDS patients. In many 'at-risk' individuals without evidence of AIDS, too, the test may be positive. For finding out the value of a particular test in at-risk and AIDS individuals, its sensitivity, specificity, precision and reproducibility (Appendix V) has to be calculated. A highly sensitive test for example, can be used for the purpose of screening of the donated blood. ELISA test is found to be exceedingly efficient as a single screen test, being 98.6 per cent specific and 97.3 per cent sensitive.

### Detection assays for HIV-1 or its antigens

In HIV-1 infections, the virus can usually be isolated from individuals who are positive for its antibodies. In some individuals, however, where a virus cannot be isolated, these assays of detecting viral antigens or the virion may be helpful. They are the (a) tests for measure of viral infectivity, (b) tests for the detection of viral antigens, and (c) tests for the detection of viral nucleic acid.

(a) Viral infectivity can be measured using either free virus, or virus-infected cells, co-cultured with a sensitive indicator cell. After some time, these recipient indicator cells start replicating the virus, which can be identified by the reverse transcriptase activity or by electron microscopy. However, this test is fairly slow and cumbersome.

(b) The second group of tests detect viral antigens by employing standard antibodies prepared against the virus in animals. The detection of viral antigens can be done either by immunofluorescence. radioimmunoassay or by ELISA test. These tests have their own advantages and disadvantages. Immunofluorescence test has the merit of directly detecting the antigens. It can easily pick the positive, flourescing-jackpot-cell. It can also locate the antigens within the cells. However, it shows a high incidence of cross-reactivity, and may also have ambiguous end points. Radioimmunoassay, similar to that employed in the antibody detection, can detect only one antigen. Nevertheless, it is fairly rapid and simple. ELISA test, on the other hand, can detect any reactive antigen.

The antigens, nevertheless, should be in substantial amount or they may escape detection, making this test less sensitive.

(c) The tests for viral nucleic acid include Southern blotting or *in situ* hybridization tests. The Southern blotting test is time-consuming, needs cloned virus probes, and requires adequate number of cells. If, however, only a few cells are at disposal, an *in situ* hybridization test may be employed, which can pick up viral DNA in 'jackpot' cells.

## OTHER LABORATORY PARAMETERS

The salient laboratory abnormalities in AIDS and pre-AIDS have been discussed elsewhere. Amongst the characteristic immunological dysfunctions, the gross paucity of $T_4$ lymphocytes heads the table. This is directly proportional to the severity of AIDS. Accordingly, there is a reversal of $T_4$ (helper/inducer) and $T_8$ (suppressor/cytotoxic) lymphocyte ratio. The *in vitro* phenotypic markers also demonstrate an overall lymphopenia. In addition, an *in vitro* functional impairment can be elicited by the phytohaemagglutinin stimulation, poke-weed mitogen, NK cytotoxicity, MLC reactivity and monocyte chemotaxis/cytotoxicity. Further, an *in vivo* functional impairment is also a feature of these patients. It is indicated by a delayed cutaneous hypersensitivity, antibody responses following immunization and the aberrant reticuloendothelial function. Serological abnormalities, too, are a prominent finding, and are constituted by hypergammaglobulinaemia, elevated levels of alpha-1 thymosine, alpha interferon, beta-2 microglobulin, antibodies to Epstein-Barr and cytomegalovirus, and also the demonstration of lymphocytotoxic antibodies.

## HISTOPATHOLOGIC MARKERS

The lymphadenopathy syndrome patients show certain distinct histopathological changes in their lymphnodes (chapter 6). Incriminating changes may also seen in the bone-marrow and lymphoid elements of the gastrointestinal tract. Electron-microscopy should be undertaken for the demonstration of HIV-1 viral inclusions. Test-tube shaped, ring-shaped and tubuloreticular inclusions, and also vesicular rosettes may also be pathognomonic of AIDS.

## RADIOLOGICAL MARKERS

The radiology may not give a clue to AIDS, unless there is a secondary development of infectious or neoplastic complications. However, AIDS patients, sooner or later, do develop these aberrations. The first and the foremost are pulmonary complications caused chiefly due to *Pneumocytis carinii*. The earliest visible radiological change is peribronchial and perivascular cuffing. Later on, diffuse reticulogranular infiltrates develop, which extend out from hilar region, often sparing the periphery. The terminal stage reveals a massively consolidated, airless lung. Other radiological change in lungs are focal/asymmetric consolidation and pleural effusion caused by *M. tuberculosis*, cavitating opacities caused by *M. tuberculosis, M. avium-intercellulare* or fungi, coarse nodular opacities of Kaposi's sarcoma, and hilar and mediastinal opacities due to Kaposi's sarcoma and lymphomas.

The CT scans of central nervous system may reveal either focal or generalized abnormalities. Focal aberrations may be caused by a variety of opportunistic infections. Multiple lesions with surrounding oedema, involving the grey/white matter interphase or basal ganglia indicate cerebral toxoplasmosis or lymphomas; progressive multifocal leucoencephalopathy shows destructive hypodense lesions confined to the superficial and deep white matter of cerebral hemispheres, having lack of contrast enhancement and absence of mass effect. The generalised abnormalities may be seen in cryptococcal meningitis, exhibiting as diffuse low-density changes in the periventricular white matter.

The clues to the gastrointestinal disease can also be picked up during radiological investigations. Typical fine ulcerations and plaques of *Candida* can be discovered in distal oesophagus on barium swallow, which can also be employed for monitoring the response to the therapy. A similar picture is produced by herpes simplex. Cytomegalovirus infection of oesophagus, on the other hand,produces a solitary large ulcer, albeit rarely. Kaposi's sarcoma lesions produce 3 to 30 mm intraluminal or intramural polypoid lesions, with central collection of barium representing ulceration. In patients with protracted, watery diarrhoea, a barium meal and follow-through reveal abnormalities of the small bowel with thickening of the mucosal folds and flocculation of barium. Oesophagoscopy, sigmoidoscopy, ultrasound and computed tomography can be used as important investigating adjuvants for the diagnosis for gastrointestinal disease.

In summary, the opportunistic infections and malignancies require their respective diagnostic procedures which when positive further add to the diagnosis of AIDS.

# 11

# Treatment

The treatment approach for an HIV patient involves inhibiting the replication of the virus using antiretroviral drugs, treatment/prophylaxis of the opportunistic infections/Malignancies and psychosocial support. Prior to the advent of antiretroviral drugs other possible modes of therapy had been *in vogue* in HIV patients (table 11.1).

**Table 11.1: Possible Modes of Therapy**

| | |
|---|---|
| Prevent Viral Entry to Cell | 1. Receptor blocker<br>2. Neutralizing antibody<br>3. Block endocytosis |
| Inhibit Viral Replication | 1. Reverse transcriptase inhibitors<br>2. Transcription of viral DNA<br>3. Cellular DNA polymerase inhibitors<br>4. Block viral protein synthesis<br>5. Block exocytosis with alpha interferon |
| Augment Immune Cell Function | 1. Thymic hormones<br>2. Lymphokines<br>3. Bone marrow transplantation<br>4. Immunomodulators |

## INTERFERONS

The biologic properties of interferons, a group of mammalian glycoproteins, include inhibition of viral replication and cellular proliferation, immunomodulation, and increase in expression of certain cell-surface antigens. In the sera of AIDS patients, elevated levels of interferon have been observed, and are seen to be associated with a poor prognosis. Moreover, a particular species of interferon, the acid-labile form has been found to appear in high-risk group at the onset of clinical AIDS. It too correlates with a poor prognosis. Other studies have demonstrated that AIDS lymphocytes make a low quantity of gamma interferon, a type of interferon known to stimulate antibody production. Further, patients with opportunistic infections show an impaired ability to produce alpha interferon.

## Alpha Interferon

The role of alpha interferon has already been shown in lymphoma, multiple myeloma, breast cancer, renal-cell carcinoma and melanoma. It has also been tested in AIDS, in both natural and recombinant forms. Trials of human lymphoblastoid alpha interferon, using daily dosage of 7.5-15 million units/$M^2$ body surface area for 28 to 60 days, have shown encouraging results. The response was more favourable in patients who had a higher total lymphocytes and $OKT_4$ cells, without opportunistic infections. The presence of endogenous acid-labile alpha interferon as well as very low $OKT_4$ cells were, however, associated with a poor response to therapy. Low or high-dose recombinant alpha-2 interferon, administered as 15 million units/$M^2$ subcutaneously, for 5 days every other week for a total of 4 cycles, also showed promising results. Both high and low dose therapy were effective, the former being more so. However, high dose therapy had a mild haematologic and systemic toxicity. Elevated interferon levels prior to treatment are usually associated with a poor response. During therapy, some augmentation of NK activity has been observed. Alpha interferons have been found to be useful in patients with Kaposi's sarcoma. Moreover, the responders did not show any increase in incidence of infectious complications, suggesting that the immune depression by interferon is not a prominent components. The recombinant preparations are tolerated better than the natural ones, and thus a higher dose can be administered.

## Gamma Interferon

It has been considered to be potentially effective in AIDS because of its capability to augment antibody production by acting as one of the direct B-cell maturing lymphokines, and its property of increasing the macrophage tumoricidal activity of stimulated *in vitro* cultures. AIDS-lymphocytes exhibit limitations in producing it *in vitro* when challenged with microbial antigens. Both natural and recombinant forms have been experimented in AIDS. Natural gamma interferon, used in the dosage of

0.1 to 10 million units/M$^2$ intramuscularly or intravenously for 5 days for 2 weeks or more has however shown no or minimal response in AIDS patients with Kaposi's sarcoma. Recombinant gamma interferon, on the other hand, has shown encouraging results when used in the dosage of 1 to 10 million units/$M_2$ twice a week by continuous intravenous infusion. Immunological parameters have demonstrated increased NK activity and augmented phytohaemagglutinin response.

**Table 11.2: Interferons in AIDS**

| Interferon | Dose | Effect |
|---|---|---|
| Alpha-2 interferon | 15 million units/M$^2$ IV or 1 million units/M$^2$ SC for 5 days, alternate week for 4 cycles | 1) Augments NK activity<br>2) Useful in Kaposi's sarcoma |
| Gamma interferon | 1-10 million units/M$^2$ twice a week by IV infusion | 1) Augments antibody production<br>2) Increases macrophage tumoricidal activity<br>3) Augments NK activity |

## INTERLEUKIN-2 STUDIES

The correction of the immunological deficit by interleukin-2 has been observed in experimental animals, where immunodeficiency was iatrogenically produced by prolonged administration of cytotoxic agents. Other evidence of immunocorrection by this agent have been observed in the form of rejection of cardiac allografts in irradiated rats. These instances have, thus, conclusively proved the role of interleukin-2 both *in vivo* and *in vitro* in reversing the immunosuppression. It is a glycoprotein of molecular weight 15,000 daltons, produced by T-lymphocytes after mitogenic or antigenic stimulation. This lymphokine is believed to get bound to a highly specific cellular receptor and effect the proliferation and expansion of activated T-cells, which in turn become cytotoxic for both alogenic and autologous fresh tumour cells (lymphokine-activated killer cell phenomenon). It also augments the production of gamma interferon by human T-cells, NK-cell activity and virus-specific cytotoxicity.

Interleukin-2 has been used in either natural or recombinant form. It is given as 24,000 to one million units/M$^2$ weekly for a total of 4 weeks. The response in AIDS patient, however, has generally been unsatisfactory.

Recombinant interleukin-2, on the other hand, holds some promise. It has to be given in high doses of either 1 million units/kg body weight by bolus infusion or as 3,000 to 10,000 units/kg/hr by continuous infusion. It has a fairly brief half-life (7-10 minutes). Its acute toxicity manifests as fever, chills, malaise, anorexia, weight gain and hepatopathy. The limitations of interleukin-2 in the management of AIDS patients include the inability of researchers to eliminate the continued presence of HIV-1 in their body, thus making the immune reconstitution only temporary.

## PHARMACOLOGIC IMMUNOMODULATORS

Certain pharmacologic agents have been observed to influence the immune system of human body. They are azimexon, bestatin, cimetidine, isoprinosine, lentinan, tuftsin, aspirin, indomethacin and levamisole. Prior to the availability of antiretroviral drugs, these agents have been tried with variable claims.

## ADOPTIVE IMMUNOTHERAPY

This forms a reasonable approach to the management of AIDS patients, as it employs measures to replace the lost T-lymphocytes. This may prove as a major breakthrough if it is promptly followed by the other immunomodulatory approaches described *vide supra,* because the previously recounted agents have apparently failed due to acute paucity of $T_4$ lymphocytes that are obviously required for the stimulation by these substances. The means incorporated in adoptive immunotherapy include lymphocyte transfusion, bone marrow transplant and thymic transplant. The result have been variable, but long term benefits are still at large. After the development of opportunistic infections or Kaposi's sarcoma, bone marrow transplants are generally ineffective. These people also fail to respond to repeated transfusions of $2 \times 10^9$ lymphocytes, although may show an initial transient modulation of immune functions. These failures appear primarily due to the continued presence of the AIDS-virus in these patients, which promptly infect the transfused cells or transplanted marrow.

The idea of thymic transplant is based on the observations that there is a profound T-cell defect in AIDS, and also there is a premature involution of thymocytes and thymic epithelium. Thymic tissue, obtained from children less than 5 years of age when undergoing cardiac surgery, was cultured for 16 days and transplanted into the muscle belly in the forearm of the AIDS patients. This brought a dramatic improvement in many of them with opportunistic infections, who got rid of these infections. An improvement of the immunological parameters was also recorded, which persisted for a variable period of time. However, the non-eradicability, as yet, of HIV-1 virus seriously reflect on these improvements.

Recently, speculative approach of adoptive immunotherapy is the treatment of AIDS patients with cultured autologous and haplo-identical lymphoid cells. Although culture of T-cells, at present, is fairly easy, yet the exactly matched lymphocytes for a particular patient are difficult to obtain.

## THYMIC HORMONES/FACTORS

Thymosin fraction 5 and thymopentin are the two major thymic hormones, whose role is being investigated in AIDS patients. In order to be effective, they required a responsive pre-T-cell population and an ability to clear HIV infection, Thymosin fraction 5 is given 30 to 120 mg daily through subcutaneous route for a period of 10 weeks. A variable immunologic modulation has been recorded. Pain and swelling at the injection site can occur at a higher doses. Thymopentin has been tried at a dosage of 15 mg intravenously three times a week for 6 weeks, but failed to evoke any response.

## OTHER IMMUNOLOGIC APPROACHES

Plasmapharesis, plasma exchange, red-cell transfusion and administration of gamma globulin or transfer factor are certain other immunologic interventions advocated in AIDS. Plasmapharesis and plasma exchange have been employed to sieve out the circulating immune complexes and also certain putative suppressor factors. Plasmapharesis with 50 ml/kg of plasma exchanged twice a week every two weeks has ushered in a transient increase in $OKT_4$ cells and mitogenic responses.

The observation that most of the infant deaths from AIDS are secondary to Gram-negative sepsis, prompted many workers to administer gamma globulin. It is given as 50-300 ml/kg every 1 to 3 weeks. Some improvement in the symptoms and a decrease in opportunistic and bacterial infections was recorded.

Transfer factor, prepared from the peripheral blood mononuclear cells, has also been employed for the management of AIDS patients. However, no response has been observed in these trials.

## ANTI RETROVIRAL THERAPY

Antiretroviral drugs work by inhibiting the multiplication of the virus. Currently available drugs generally target 2 key enzymes that the virus requires in order to replicate: protease and reverse transcriptase. Thus, protease inhibitors (PIs) inhibit the protease enzyme, whereas reverse transcriptase inhibitors inhibit the reverse transcriptase enzyme. Reverse transcriptase inhibitors are further divided into two types – nucleoside reverse transcriptase inhibitors (NRTIs) and non-nucleoside reverse transcriptase inhibitors (NNRTIs) – based on slight differences in their chemical structure and mode of action. (Table 11.3).

The 2001 Guidelines for the use of antiretroviral agents have been well-established. Current combination therapy for HIV infection is complex for both the doctor and patient. Highly active antiretroviral therapy (HAART) is defined as three or more antiretroviral drugs from two or three different classes of drugs. Initiating therapy, combining drug classes, negotiating treatment regimens, and monitoring laboratory parameters are complex tasks requiring an HIV expert.

**Table 11.3: Classes of antiretrovirals**

| Nucleoside Reverse Transcriptase Inhibitors (NRTIs) | Non-Nucleoside Reverse Transcriptase Inhibitors (NNRTIs) | Protease Inhibitors (PIs) |
|---|---|---|
| Zidovudine | Nevirapine | Indinavir |
| Stavudine | Efavirenz | Nelfinavir |
| Lamivudine | Delavirdine | Ritonavir |
| Didanosine | | Saquinavir |
| Zalcitabine | | Amprenavir |
| Abacavir | | Lopinavir/Ritonavir |
| Combivir | | |
| Trizivir | | |

Therapy with antiretroviral agents is recommended for all HIV patients with acute HIV syndrome, patients within 6 months of seroconversion, any symptomatic HIV-positive patient, postexposure prophylaxis, and pregnant women to prevent vertical transmission. Acute treatment of a serious opportunistic infection takes precedence over antiretroviral therapy. Before commencing antiretroviral therapy, it is important to discuss the following points with the patient:

1. Therapy is not curative

2. Treatment is lifelong
3. Cost of therapy and follow-up should be taken into account
4. Long-term adverse events may occur with antiretroviral therapy
5. Pill burden i.e. a number of medications have to be taken daily as prescribed.
6. Adherence is critical
7. Even if a patient is responding well to therapy, he is still infectious and capable of transmitting the virus. Hence, safer sex should be practiced.

The HAART regimens may include combinations of one or more of a nucleoside reverse transcriptase inhibitor (NRTI), non-nucleoside reverse transcriptase inhibitor (NNRTI), and protease inhibitor (PI). Various combinations are possible, based upon clinical trials that determine efficacy, adverse effects, interactions, and ease of use. The standard recommended regimens are as follows:

- NRTI + NRTI + PI
- NRTI + NRTI + NNRTI
- NRTI + NRTI + PI + PI

While choosing the 2-NRTI component, the following two-NRTI combinations are **contraindicated:**

1. Zidovudine + stavudine
2. Zalcitabine + stavudine
3. Zalcitabine + didanosine

The disadvantage of HAART therapy is that antiretroviral agents are not virucidal, thus eradication with these drug cocktails cannot be achieved. When HAART therapy is stopped, viral loads return to pre-treatment levels. New drug classes under investigation may completely prevent fusion between the HIV virus and healthy cells.

Table 11.4 (a, b and c) have reviewed the present antiretrorival drugs along with salient features.

Three new drugs have become available for use in treatment failure.

(a) **Enfuvirtide.** A subcutaneously administered HIV fusion inhibitor, enfuvirtide was evaluated in 2 large phase 3 trials in patients with advanced HIV disease (median CD4 cell count, 90/μL); in patients with multiple previous and current treatment failures (median, 12 prior antiretroviral drugs); and in patients with a median HIV RNA level of 130000 copies/mL. Patients were randomized to receive an optimized

**Table 11.4a: Nucleoside Reverse Transcriptase inhibitors (NRTIs) (Carrasco and Tyring, 2001)**

| Drug | Form | Dose | Dietary | Adverse Events | Labs |
|---|---|---|---|---|---|
| Zidovudine (Retrovir) AZT | 100 mg caps<br>300 mg tabs<br>10 mg/mL IV solution<br>10 mg/mL oral solution | 200 mg TID<br>300 mg BID | None | Bone marrow suppression: anemia or neutropenia<br>GI: nausea, vomiting, hepatotoxicity, hapatic steatosis<br>Others: fatigue, metabolic acidosis, myopathy, myositis, headache, insomnia, hyperpigmented and slow-growing nails, uritcaria, pruritus, nonspecific maculopapular rash | CBC<br>electrolytes<br>CK<br>LFTs |
| Lamivudine (Epivir) 3TC | 150 mg tabs<br>10 mg/mL solution | 150 mg BID | None | Nausea, vomiting, anorexia, lactic acidosis, hepatic steatosis peripheral neuropathy, headache, malaise, pancreatitis, hyperglycemia, fatigue psychosis, and mania | amylase<br>lipase |
| Stavudine (Zerit) D4T | 15 mg caps<br>20 mg caps<br>30 mg caps<br>40 mg caps<br>1 mg/mL solution | 40 mg BID | None | Peripheral neuropathy, lactic acidosis<br>Hepatic steatosis, myopathy, and pancreatitis | amylase<br>lipase<br>LFTs |
| Didanosine (Videx) DdI | 25 mg tabs<br>50 mg tabs<br>100 mg tabs<br>150 mg tabs<br>200 mg tabs<br>167 mg sachets | 200 mg Tabs BID<br>250 mg Powder BID<br>400 mg Tabs | 30 min before meals | Nausea, vomiting, diarrhea, peripheral neuropathy, pancreatitis, hepatitis, lactic acidosis with hepatic steatosis, dry mouth, hypertriglyceridemia, hyperuricemia, optic neuritis, | amylase<br>lipase<br>LFTs<br>lipids |

(Contd.)

| Drug | Form | Dose | Dietary | Adverse Events | Labs |
|---|---|---|---|---|---|
| | 250 mg sachets<br>400 m EC caps. | qd | | and rash | |
| Zalcitabine (Hivid) ddC | 0.375 mg tabs<br>0.75 mg tabs | 0.75 mg TID | Avoid aluminium & magnesium antacids | Peripheral neuropathy, neutropenia, pancreatitis, aphthous ulcers, stomatitis, esophageal ulcers, hepatomegaly, steatosis, lactic acidosis, reported urticaria, and one anaphylactoid reaction | CBC<br>amylase<br>lipase |
| Abacavir (Ziagen) ABC | 300 mg tabs<br>20 mg/mL solution | 300 mg BID | None; avoid alcohol | Hypersensitivity syndrome, fever, maculopapular rash, nausea, vomiting, fatigue, diarrhea, anorexia, malaise, myalgias, arthralgias, lactic acidosis with hepatic steatosis, hepatitis, respiratory symptoms such as sore throat, cough, and shortness of breath | Amylase<br>lipase<br>CK<br>LFT's |
| Combivir | 300 mg AZT<br>150 mg 3TC | BID | None | As above | CBC<br>electrolytes<br>CK LFTs<br>amylase<br>lipase |
| Trizivir | 300 mg AZT<br>150 mg 3TC<br>300 mg ABC | BID | None | As above | CBC<br>electrolytes<br>CK LFTs<br>amylase<br>lipase |

**Table 11.4b: Non-Nucleoside Reverse Transcriptase Inhibitors (NNRTIs) (Carrasco and Tyring, 2001)**

| Drug | Form | Dose | Dietary | Adverse Events | Labs |
|---|---|---|---|---|---|
| Nevirapine (Viramune) | 200-mg tabs 50-mg/5 mL susp | 200 mg × 14d then 200 mg BID | None | Rash, Stevens-Johnson Syndrome and Hepatitis | LFTs |
| Delavirdine (Rescriptor) | 100-mg tabs 200-mg tabs | 400 mg TID four 100 mg tabs dissolve in 3 oz water TID | 1 hour apart from antacids, no regard to meals | Rash, Stevens-Johnson Syndrome, Hapatitis, headaches, increased LFTs | LFTs |
| Efavirenz (Sustiva) | 50-mg caps 100-mg caps 200-mg caps | 600 mg qhs | Avoid high-fat meals | Dizziness, insomnia, nightmares, delusions, hallucinations, amnesia, confusion, impaired concentration, somnolence, agitation, euphoria, depersonalization, depression, maculpapular rash, increased LFTs, false-positive cannabinoid test | LFTs |

**Table 11.4c: Protease Inhibitors (PIs) (Carrasco and Tyring, 2001)**

| Drug | Form | Dose | Dietary | Adverse Events | Labs |
|---|---|---|---|---|---|
| Saquinavir (Fortovase) (Invirase) | 200-mg caps soft gel 200-mg caps hard gel | 1200 mg TID soft gel 400 mg TID hard gel | With food (within 2 hours of a meal) | Nausea, vomiting, diarrhea, hepatitis, lipodystrophy, hyperlipidemia, diabetes mellitus, hyperglycemia, headache, elevated LFTs, abnormal fat distribution (lipodystrophy) | LFTs Lipids glucose |
| Ritonavir (Norvir) | 100-mg caps 600-mg/7.5 mL soln. | 600 mg BID or 7.5 mL BID | With food refrigerate caps not soln | Nausea, vomiting, diarrhea, hepatitis, pancreatitis, hyperlipidemia, hyperglycemia, peripheral neuropathy, circumoral paraesthesias, asthenia, abnormal fat distribution, unpalatable taste, maculopapular rash, increased CK, uric acid, and LFTs | LFTs lipids amylase lipase glucose |
| Indinavir (Crixivan) | 200-mg caps 333-mg caps 400-mg caps | 800 mg q8h separate dosing with ddl by 1 h. | With food (1h before or 2h after meals) Drink plenty of water | Nausea, vomiting, diarrhea, hepatitis, nephrolithiasis, acute interstitial nephritis, acute renal failure, hyperglycemia, diabetes mellitus, hyperlipidemia, hemolysis, thrombocytopenia, rash, abnormal fat distribution, headache, asthenia, blurred vision, dizziness, and metallic taste | LFTs lipids glucose UA Creat. |

*(Contd.)*

| Drug | Form | Dose | Dietary | Adverse Events | Labs |
|---|---|---|---|---|---|
| Nelfinavir (Viracept) | 250-mg tabs 50-mg/g powder | 750 mg TID 1250 mg BID | With food | Diarrhea, hepatitis, hyperlipidemia, hyperglycemia, and abnormal fat redistribution | LFTs lipids glucose |
| Amprenavir (Agenerase) | 50-mg caps 150-mg caps 15-mg/mL soln. | 1200 mg BID 1400 mg BID soln. | Avoid high-fat meals | Nausea, vomiting, diarrhea, hepatitis, circumoral paraesthesias, hyperlipidemias, diabetes mellitus, hemolytic anemia, rash, lipodystrophy | LFTs amylase lipase glucose |
| Lopinavir + ritonavir (Kaletra) | 133.3 mg lopinavir +33.3 mg ritonavir 400 mg lopinavir +100 mg ritonavir (solution) in 5 mL | 400 mg lopinavir +100 mg ritonavir BID | with food | Nausea, vomiting, diarrhea, asthenia, increased transaminases, hyperglycemia, lipodystrophy, hyperlipidemia | LFTs Lipids amylase glucose lipase |

background therapy with or without the addition of enfuvirtide. After 48 weeks, the enfuvirtide group had a significantly greater decrease in HIV RNA level (1.48 $\log_{10}$ reduction) than the optimized background only group (0.63 $\log_{10}$ reduction). With the exception of frequent injection-site reactions, the durg was well tolerated.

(b) **Atazanavir.** A regimen containing 300 mg/d of atazanavir and 100 mg/d of ritonavir provided viral load reduction at 24 weeks comparable to lopinavir/ritonavir, whereas 40 mg/d of atazanavir (unboosted) was inferior to lopinavir/ritonavir. The combination of atazanavir and low dose ritonavir was associated with less elevation of plasma lipid levels than boosted protease inhibitor comparators in treatment experienced patients. Tenofovir coadministration diminishes the oral bio-availability of atazanavir.

(c) **Fosamprenavir.** A prodrug of amprenavir, fosamprenavir has higher bioavailability and an improved formulation over the parent compound. Fosamprenavir should be administered with low-dose ritonavir (700 mg of fosamprenavir and 100 mg of ritonavir twice daily) (evidence strength rating, IB). In a comparative study, fosamprenavir with low-dose ritonavir taken twice daily had similar activity and tolerability as lopinavir/ritonavir.

## Post-exposure prophylaxis (PEP) of health-care workers

Healthcare workers (HCWs) whose activities involve contact with HIV-infected patients, or who may come in contact with blood or body fluid from HIV-positive patients in a health care or laboratory setting are at risk for occupational exposure to HIV.

The centers for Disease Control (CDC) based at Atlanta, USA, has issued guidelines for treatment of occupational exposure to HIV (also referred to as 'post-exposure prophylaxis' or PEP). The rationale behind PEP is that antiretroviral treatment started immediately after exposure to HIV may abort infection by inhibiting HIV replication (Fig. 11.1). If PEP is indicated, it should be started within 1 to 2 hours of exposure with the recommended regimen (Table 11.5).

**Table 11.5: Recommended regimen for post-exposure prophylaxis**

| Category | Drug regimen |
|---|---|
| Basic | Zidovudine 300 mg bid + Lamivudine 150 mg bid for 28 days |
| Expanded | Basic regimen + indinavir 800 mg tid or nelfinavir 750 mg tid for 28 days |

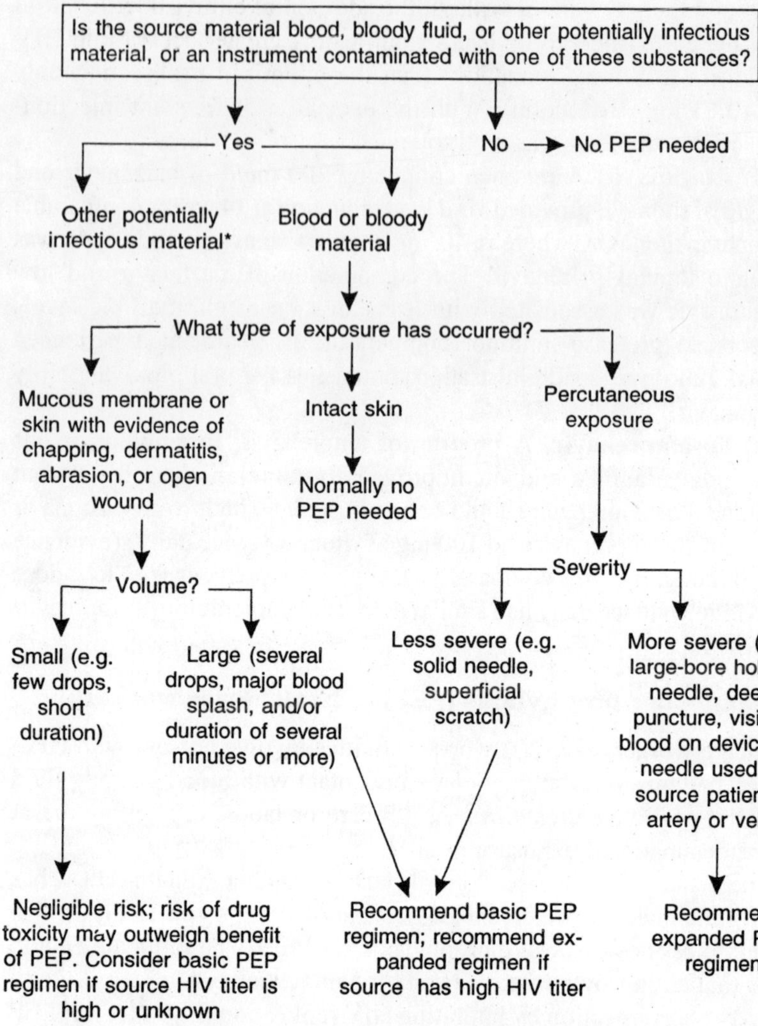


* Other potentially infectious materials include semen; vaginal secretions; cerebrospinal, synovial, pleural, peritoneal, pericardial, or amniotic fluids, or tissue. These body substances generally carry a low risk of infection in health care settings.

**Fig. 11.1. Post exposure prophylaxis for HCWs**

## Limitations of Antiretroviral therapy

1. *Drug interactions:* Drug interactions of antiretroviral drugs with other medications required for opportunistic infections and

malignancies pose a serious limitation on the latter's use concomitantly (Table 11.6).

**Table 11.6: Potential Drug Interactions with Antiretroviral Medications**

| Antiretroviral Medication for HIV/AIDS | Potential Drug Interaction with |
|---|---|
| ***Nucleoside reverse transcriptase inhibitors*** | |
| Lamivudine (3TC) | TMP-SMX, Aminoglycosides, Amphotericin B |
| Zalcitabine (ddC) | Cimetidine, Foscarnet, Magnesium/Aluminium antacids, Peripheral neuropathy-causing agents |
| Zidovudine (AZT) | Acetaminophen, Acyclovir, Amphotericin B, Aspirin, Cimetidine, Clarithromycin, Dapsone, Erythromycin, Fluconazole, Ganciclovir, Ibuprofen, Indomethacin, Interferon, Ketoconazole, Phenytoin, PUVA, TMA-SMX |
| Didanosine (ddl) | Amphotericin B, Azathioprine, Cimetidine, Corticosteroids, Dapsone, Intraconazole, Ketoconazole, Mercaptopurine, Phenytoin, Quinolones, Tetracycline, TMP-SMX |
| Stavudine (d4T) | Amphotericin B, Peripheral neuropathy-causing agents |
| Abacavir | Ethanol |
| ***Protease inhibitors*** | |
| Indinavir | Astemizole, Benzodiazepines, Clarithromycin, Cyclosporine, Fluconazole, Itraconazole, Ketoconazole, Rifamycins, Terfenadine |
| Saquinavir | Astemizole, Benzodiazepines, Clindamycin, Cyclosporine, Dapsone, Fluconazole, Ketoconazole, Phenytoin, PUVA, Terfenadine |
| Ritonavir | Astemizole, Benzodiazepines, Chloroquine, Cimetidine, Clarithromycin, Codeine, Cyclophosphamide, Cyclosporine, Erythromycin, Fluconazole, Ibuprofen, Indomethacin, Itraconazole, Ketoconazole, Lidocaine, Loratidine, Meperidine, Metronidazole, Morphine, Pentoxyfylline, Prednisone, Primaquine, Propoxyphene, Rifamycins, Tacrolimus |
| Nelfinavir | Terfenadine, Tricyclic antidepressants, Benzodiazepines, Cyclosporine, Fluconazole, Ketoconazole |

*(Contd.)*

| Antiretroviral Medication for HIV/AIDS | Potential Drug Interaction with |
|---|---|
| ***Nonnucleoside reverse transcriptase inhibitors*** | |
| Delavirdine mesylate | Astemizole,Benzodiazepines, Climetidine, Clarithromycin, Dapsone, Ketaconazole, Rifamycins, Terfenadine |
| Nevirapine | Rifamycins |
| Efavirenz | Rifamycins, Clarithromycin, Estrogens |

2. *Adherence:* Due to several restrictions in diet as well as side-effects, the patients find it difficult to adhere especially due to a prolonged therapy.
3. *Long term complications:* Lipodystrophy, hypertension, hyperlipidemia, diabetes, osteoporosis, gynaecomastia, renal damage and calculi and myocardial infarction all are serious side effects.
4. *Cost:* A prolonged treatment with costly medicines puts pressure on already demoralized patent.

## THERAPY OF INFECTIONS COMPLICATIONS

### A. Protozoal infections

***Pneumocystis carinii infections:*** The drugs of choice are cotrimoxazole (Trimethoprim-sulfamethoxazole) and pentamidine isethionate. Cotrimoxazole is given upto 20 mg per kilogram body weight daily of trimethoprim component, in 3 or 4 divided oral doses, or intravenously, given for 3 weeks or more depending upon the clinical response, and for preventing relapse. The dose has to be proportionately reduced in patients with impaired renal functions. The AIDS patients on this therapy, for reasons hitherto ambiguous, show a high incidence (65%) of side-effects including rash, drug fever and leukopenia. If the clinical condition of the patient does not improve even after 5 days of therapy, pentamidine may be added. Cotrimoxazole can also be used for chemoprophylaxis in AIDS patients as 2.5 mg per kilogram of trimethoprim component twice daily or biweekly to patients who tolerate it well. Sulfidoxine-pyrimethamine prophylaxis has also been tried with variable success.

Pentamidine isethionate is administered as 4 mg per kilogram of body weight daily by intramuscular route. It is sometimes given in combination or substituted for cotrimoxazole, if latter does not give adequate response or can not be tolerated. The common side-effects of pentamidine include nephrotoxicity, thrombocytopenia, sterile abscesses

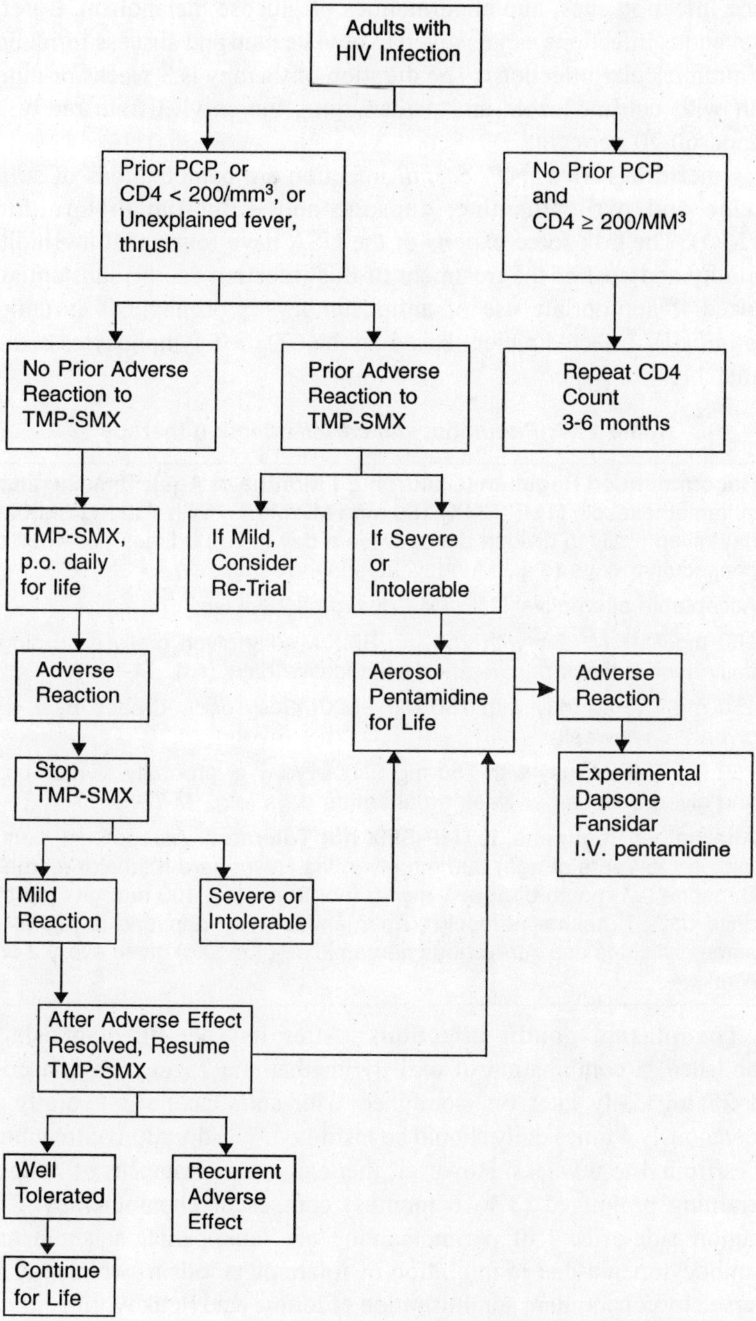


**Fig. 11.2. Recommendations on Antipneumocystis Prophylaxis**
(Courtesy MMWR, 1992)

at the infection sites, and abnormalities of glucose metabolism. Careful intravenous infections can be given to obviate pain and abscess formation by intramuscular infections. The duration of therapy is 3 weeks or more. Both with cotrimoxazole and pentamidine, the survival rate rarely go beyond 60-70 per cent.

Other drugs tried in *P. carinii* infection are combinations of sulfadiazine and pyrimethamine, dapsone and difluoromethylornithine (DFMO). The task force experts of the USA have found that morbidity, mortality and cost of the treatment of this infection can be substantially reduced if appropriate use of antipneumocystis prophylaxis is undertaken in HIV-infected patient based on the $CD_4$ + T-lymphocytes counts (Table 11.7).

**Table 11.7: *Pneumocystis carinii* infection therapy**

I. **Recommended Regimen (Children ≥ 1 Months of Age):** Trimethoprium/sulfamethoxazole (TMP-SMX) 150 mg TMP/M$^2$/day with 750 mg SMX/M$^2$/day given orally in divided doses twice a day (b.i.d.) 3 times per week on consecutive days (e.g., Monday-Tuesday-Wednesday)

   Acceptable alternative TMP/SMX dosage schedules:

A. 150 mg TMP/M$^2$/day with 750 mg SMX/M$^2$/day given orally as a single daily dose 3 times per week on consecutive days (e.g., M-T-W)

B. 150 mg TMP/M$^2$/day with 750 mg SMX/M$^2$/day orally divided b.i.d. and given 7 days/week

C. 150 mg TMP/M$^2$/day with 750 mg SNX/M$^2$/day given orally divided b.i.d. and given 3 times per week on alternate days (e.g., M-W-F)

II. **Alternative Regimens, If TMP-SMX not Tolerated:** Aerosolized pentamidine (≥5 years of age) 300 mg given via Respirgard II inhaler monthly. Dapsone (≥1 month of age) 1 mg/kg (not to exceed 100 mg) given orally once daily. If neither aerosolized pentamidine nor dapsone is tolerated, some clinicians use intravenous pentamidine (4 mg/kg) given every 2 or 4 weeks.

**Toxoplasma gondii infections:** After its specific diagnosis is established, a combination of oral pyrimethamine 75 mg for first dose and 25 mg daily later on, combined with sulfadiazine 2 g orally or intravenously 4 times daily should be instituted. The duration of treatment varies from 4 to 6 weeks. However, there are many instances of relapse, warranting prolonged (3 to 6 months) courses of chemotherapy. The common side-effects of pyrimethamine are leukopenia, anaemia and thrombocytopenia due to inhibition of folate metabolism which can be reversed by concomitant administration of folinic acid (leukovorim citrate)

2 to 3 times every week orally or 10 mg by intravenous route. Other side-effects attributed to this combination are skin rash and abnormalities of liver functions.

The alternative drugs for toxoplasmosis are oral clindamycin 300 to 450 mg four times daily, and spiramycin 50 mg per kilogram body weight daily in 2-4 divided doses.

**Cryptosporidium infections:** This protozoa has till date defied a successful treament. In non-AIDS patients, on immunosuppressive therapy, this infection can be cleared by reducing the dose of these agents. The AIDS patients, however, have proved futile any attempt of immuno-modulation. The drug currently advocated for this infection is spiramycin 1g, 3 times daily for a duration varying from one to 16 weeks. The side-effects include nausea, vomiting, diarrhoea, epigastric pain, and acute colitis. In addition to spiramycin, antidiarrhoeal agents and nutritional supplements should also be administered.

## B. Fungal Infections

**Candidiasis:** The treatment of candidiasis in fairly easy. However, AIDS patient usually relapse once the therapy is stopped. Oral thrush can be treated with nystatin 400,000 units or clotrimazole troches given every 4 hourly. More extensive lesions require oral Ketoconazole 200 mg twice daily, or amphotericin-B 0.3 to 0.6 mg/kg daily for 5 to 7 days. The relapses require a maintenance doses of nystatin, clotrimazole or keto-conazole.

**Cryptococcosis:** All patients showing positive cultures should be energetically treated, as it shows a high incidence of dissemination. Amphotericin-B 0.3 mg per kilogram of body weight combined with 150 mg/kg of flucytosine daily should be given for a period of 5-6 weeks. Flucytosine can cause progressive, severe leukopenia, and thus may have to be withdrawn in many patients. Alternatively, amphotericin may be given alone as 0.6 mg/kg/day for 10 weeks. Relapses are, however, common, requiring repeated courses of chemotherapy. Moreover, cryptococcal antigen titres, and occasionally cultures may remain positive despite successful therapy.

## C. Bacterial Infections

**Mycobacterium avium-intracellulare:** The management of this myco-bacteria is pretty difficult as it is resistant to conventional antitubercular chemotherapeutic agents. In one study, the National Institute of Health,

U.S.A. cultured 31 isolates, of which only 3% were susceptible to 1.0 μg/ml of isoniazid, 12% to 5.0μg/ml of isoniazid, 66% to 10 μg/ml of ehthambutol, 6% to 1.0 μg/ml of rifampicin, and 12% to 5.0 μg/ml of rifampicin. Two experimental drugs, however, have shown promising results. They are ansaymcin and clofazimine, given in the daily dosage of 150-300 mg. and 100-500 mg respectively.

Public health service, USA recommends that every regimen should contain either azithromycin or clarithromycin. A life-long regimen combining clarithromycin 500 mg PO BID with ethambutol 15-20 mg/kg/d ± rifabutin 300 mg PO QD is generally effective. Azithromycin can be used in patients who are intolerant of clarithromycin. Many experts prefer ethambutol as a second drug. Some clinicians have added one or more of the following as second, third, for fourth agents: clofazimine, rifabutin, rifampin, ciprofloxacin, and in some situations amikacin. Isoniazid and pyrazinamide are not effective for the therapy of *Mycobacterium avium*-complex (MAC).

Clinical manifestations of disseminated MAC-such as fever, weight loss, and night sweats-should be monitored several time during the initial weeks of therapy. Microbiologic response, as assessed by blood culture every 4 weeks during initial therapy, can also be helpful in interpreting the efficiency of a therapeutic regimen. Therapy should continue for the lifetime of the patient if clinical and microbiologic improvements is observed.

Preventive therapy against MAC is recommended when the CD4 count is < 50/μl, in patients with no active disease due to MAC, TB, or any other mycobacteria. Assess potential risks/benefits individually. Prophylactic regimens include (in descending order of preference) Azithromycin 1200 mg/wk PO, or Clarithromycin 500 mg PO BID, or Rifabutin 300 mg PO QD.

**Mycobacterium tuberculosis:** The antitubercular regimens used in AIDS patients are no different than those administered in other tuberculosis patients, incorporating 3 or 4 drug regimens. However, the duration of therapy may have to be prolonged. Initial treatment with 4 drugs (INH 300 mg PO QD, rifampin 600 mg PO QD, ethambutol 15 mg/kg/d, and PZA 25 mg/kg/d) is recommended until results of culture and susceptibility are available. In areas, where INH resistance rate is > 4%, streptomycin should be added to the initial treatment regimen until susceptibility results are available. If TB isolate is fully susceptible. INH and rifampin should be continued for 9 months, or at least 6 months beyond the last positive culture. However, the optimal length of therapy for HIV-infected TB patients has not been established. It is especially important to assess the clinical and bacteriologic response when treating patients infected with HIV; treatment should be prolonged beyond 6 months if the response is slow or suboptimal. The patients are likely to relapses after cessation of the drugs. Concurrent occurrence of other infections may also pose a challenge to the treating physician, as are the increased incidence of untoward reactions of the drugs.

### D. Viral infection

**Cytomegalovirus infections:** Cytomegaloviruses themselves are immuno-suppressive, and thus facilitate the occurrence of internal malignancies. These infections should, therefore, be promptly eradicated. Paradoxically, there is no effective therapy for cytomegalovirus, although its infection is fairly common. Recently, newer drugs like DHPG or B759U have been tried with variable efficacy.

**Herpes simplex/zoster infection:** Extensive herpes simplex ulceration require 5 mg/kg of acyclovir intravenously three times daily for 1-2 weeks. In milder cases, oral cyclovir 200 mg thrice or five times daily can be administered. Recurrences are, however, common. Similarly, disseminated zoster requires intravenous acyclovir 10 mg per kg body weight three times daily. Recurrences of lesions in the same dermatomes is the rule, although it may take several weeks.

**Other viral infections:** Epsten-Barr virus infection has desisted all antiviral treatments. Molluscum contagiosa lesions require the usual treatment in the form of expression of the central cheesy material with a fine needle followed by 50 per cent trichloroacetic acid cauterization of the bleeding base. Being numerous in number, they require several shifts for complete treatment. Condyloma acuminata too have to be dealt with in the conventional way. Podophyllum resin 20% in tincture benzoin in to be carefully applied after cordoning off the surrounding area with petrolatum or protective jelly. The chemical has to be washed after 3-4 hours of application. It is usually given biweekly till be lesions regress.

## MANAGEMENT OF KAPOSI'S SARCOMA

Prior to the advent of AIDS, Kaposi's sarcoma existed as classic and African forms, and thus experience of treating the same has been applied in AIDS patients suffering from this malignancy. The problem, however, is that AIDS patients already have profound immunosuppression, making the administration of cytostatic drugs a dangerous exercise, which may result in fatal opportunistic infections. It is also well-experienced that opportunistic microbes are the prime killers of AIDS patients, rather than Kaposi's sarcoma alone. The following modalities have been used with variable success.

## Surgery and Irradiation

Early lesions of Kaposi's sarcoma which are small and localized, can easily be excised by curettage, surgical excision or electrodessication. Being a radioresponsive tumour, the lesions localised to skin or oral cavity can be excellently treated with electronbeam irradiation therapy. Radiations have also been tried with moderate success in localized bone and visceral lesions.

## Chemotherapy

An extensive, multifocal Kaposi's sarcoma, which is usual in AIDS patients, naturally warrants a combination chemotherapy. The risks of such a regimen are sometimes grave, but probably justifiable in disseminated Kaposi's sarcoma involving various organ-systems of the body. Vinblastine has been a commonly used agent, which gives a 90-95 per cent response rate in classic and African Kaposi's sarcoma. Its response rate, however, is only 20-37 per cent in AIDS-related (Epidemic) Kaposi's sarcoma, which can be increased to 50-75 per cent if AIDS-patient reports for treatment early in the course of the disease. A combination therapy constituting adreomycin, bleomycin and vinblastine (ABV) has shown no apparant superiority over vinblastine alone, but shows a high incidence of opportunistic infections. On the other hand, combination chemotherapy is very beneficial in the African type of the disease, with less side-effects.

Etoposide (VP-16-213) has also been used in this neoplasm with promising results. It is a podophyllotoxin having a relatively good subjective tolerance, and lacks cross-resistance to combination drug regimens. ABV regimen combined with dacarbazine (ABVD) has also shown encouraging response.

## Immunotherapy

Immune modulator therapy can prove invaluable, as they will prevent the development/worsening of opportunistic infections during the management of Kaposi's sarcoma. Interferons (alpha, gamma) have also been tested in AIDS patients, as they have immunomodulatory as well as antiproliferative properties. Alpha interferons have been extensively studied in epidemic Kaposi's sarcoma. They have been used either as high-dose ($50 \times 60^6$ U/

$M^2$ IV) or low-dose ($1 \times 10^6$ U/$M^2$ SC) recombinant alpha-2-interferons for 5 consecutive days every other week for 8 weeks, followed by a maintenance therapy. A high-dose therapy, however, proved more effective. Treatments are well-tolerated. Side-effects recorded are flu-like syndrome, and toxicity is minimal and comprises of reversible changes in serum transaminases levels and myelosuppression. It, however does not influence the carrier state/disease of cytomegalovirus.

Gamma (immune) interferon has also been tried. It is derived from T-lymphocytes and promotes antibody-dependent cell-mediated cytotoxicity. It also simulate the generation of natural Killer (NK) cell activity. AIDS patients have been shown to be deficient in the production of interleukin-2, and thus this agent has also been tried for reconstituting the shattered immune system of AIDS victim.

In summary, the localised or stage I Kaposi's sarcoma should be treated only with local modalities such as surgical excision or radiotherapy, while the patients with disseminated disease without B-symptoms (see chapter 8) require single-agent chemotherapy or immunomodulators. The remaining patients of Kaposi's sarcoma having disseminated, aggressive disease with visceral involvement, or with B-symptoms should receive a combination chemotherapy.

## PROSPECTS FOR A VACCINE

The constitution of a safe, immunogenic and protective vaccine against AIDS, that is capable of eliciting a neutralizing antibody response in the host, will prove invaluable in immunizing the susceptible population. It can theoretically be achieved either by using a modified avirulent virus, inactivated virus or by using viral subunits. Non-pathogenic live viruses, which are either natural variants or manufactured mutations/deletions can be worked out for the formation of vaccines, Inactivated virus, too, can serve this purpose. Other approaches to vaccine formation include the subunit vaccines that incorporates a part of the virus capable of inducing the production of neutralizing antibodies in the host, such as envelop glycoprotein or the glycoprotein-transmembrane antigen complex. Genetically engineered glycoprotein antigens can also be employed after getting them introduced in the vaccinia virus genome. And lastly, sequence-derived peptides of neutralizing epitomes or anti-idiotypes of neutralizing monoclonal antibodies can also serve as vaccines. However, it is not as simple as speculations. Researchers ploughing this aspect of therapy have met many intriguing and discouraging situations, like the observation that the fragile nature of the HIV-1 envelop makes for a poor immunogen when inactivated by formalin, and the ability of retroviruses to show genomic variations in attenuated form, which can prove catastrophic. The latter experience, thus, demands for a vaccine which lacks viral RNA.

It is well-known that AIDS patients do not develop neutralizing antibodies, and thus have no immunity against HIV-1. The viral envelop vaccines so far developed, too, chiefly induce the non-neutralizing antibodies. A low level of neutralizing antibodies, nevertheless, has been demonstrated to be raised by some recombinant envelop vaccines. Viral envelop proteins required for these trials can be procured by gently disrupting the virus, and separating out the envelop (especially the glycoprotein 120) by gradient centrifugation. The envelop protein can also be introduced into the vaccinia virus genome, which will act as a live viral vector for HIV envelop, and can also initiate the formation of neutralizing antibodies. However, no concrete success has so far been obtained in this regard. The development of an anti-idiotype is a recent advance towards as effective vaccine for AIDS. When an antibody is developed against some specific antigen, the variable region of the antibody is infact the mirror image of the antigen (epitope). It may then assume an antigenic role itself, and antibodies may generate against this region, termed as anti-idiotype antibodies. Immunologically their appearance will exactly mimic the original antigen. This is the basis of this recent vaccine. Vaccine development has encountered several obstacles: HIV epitope variability, HIV avoidance of immune response through cell to cell transmission, lack of an effective antibody response, and induction of adverse immune reactions through HIV homology to endogenous human proteins. Several vaccine strategies have been proposed, including induction of cell mediated and/or humoral immunity. The most advanced vaccine research has centered on the used of the HIV gp 120 or gp 160 envelope proteins to induce a humoral response. Most neutralizing antibodies formed in persons infected with HIV are aimed at gp 160. However, several research studies have focused on use of gp 120 because it was simpler to manufacture and did not have any major disadvantages compared to gp 160.

So far, only VaxGen, has received approval from the FDA to go ahead with the first full scale human testing of a possible AIDS vaccine. Vax Gen's product is made from tiny recombinant fragments of $gp^{120}$. As the vaccine does not contain a live HIV strain, it is safe in human beings. However, induction of antibodies by the vaccine is meagre and so it is hitherto not useful.

# 12

# Prevention Only Sure Cure

The fact that there is no effective treatment of AIDS virus and of the immunologic defects ushered in by it, as well as discouraging therapy of opportunistic infections and unusual malignancies, speaks by itself that the prevention of AIDS will prove as a major step in controlling this disease. The near-exclusive occurrence of this infection in certain high-risk individuals make this task a bit more fruitful should these groups are carefully surveyed, examined and educated.

### (a) Sexual Transmission

The changing pattern of life have resulted in certain derogatory advances in human scenario. One of its major components is the promiscuity and unnatural sexual practices including homosexual acts and bestiality. The promiscuity is on the increase because of more social freedom, easy availability of contraceptive devices and abortion facilities, prostitution, and frequent travels to anonymous places which removes social fears. Easy travel facilities all over the globe are also a chief factor of speedy transmission of infective disorders from one geographic area to another, through a human 'vector'. Thus, in escaping this dreaded scourge, the first and the foremost step is to re-establish the dishevelled threads of social conduct, and regain the old moral values. One should avoid many sexual partners, refrain from sex with strangers and forbid unnatural sexual practices including homosexuality. This will go a long way in controlling the transmission of the disease. Monogamous relationship between partners known to be uninfected is practically risk-free, as was usually practised in the past. Alternatively, they should practise 'safe sex' i.e. reduce the number of partners, avoid high risk group (drug abusers, prostitutes etc.) and use condoms.

### (b) Intravenous Drug Abusers

The intravenous drug abusers, similarly, have to be brought to the book, and guided sympathetically to abandon this habit. Still, if they are incorrigible, they should be advised to use sterile syringes and needles, without sharing, and destroy them after use.

### (c) Blood and Blood Product recipients

The people who require repeated blood/blood product infusions should be carefully monitored. Blood donation by high-risk groups should be discouraged. Blood should routinely be screened for HIV antibodies, and individual blood products should be treated by different ways i.e. heat treatment etc.

### (d) Health Care Workers

Another preventive facet of AIDS deals with the management of pre-AIDS and AIDS patients, because their body secretions are potentially infective, and may transmit the infection to innocent medical, paramedical and sanitary workers. An elaborate knowledge of these preventive measures in AIDS is mandatory for all people dealing with AIDS-patients including community workers. In addition to routine hygiene and aseptic technique, fastidious care in the handling and disposal of used sharps in essential, Care should be taken to avoid contact with patients' body fluids, especially on to broken skin or mucous membranes such as conjunctiva, thus involving more frequent use of gloves, masks and eye protection. For sterilization of instruments, heat is the most reliable method. Fresh 2% alkaline glutaraldeyde is an effective disinfectant for heat-sensitive equipment if properly used but may be irritant to the tissues. For disinfection of surfaces, sodium hypochlorite 1% (household bleach) diluted 1:10 to give 1000 ppm available chlorine is generally satisfactory. Infection control advisers will provide detailed guidance locally.

### (e) HIV-infected women and those in high-risk groups

Such individuals should practise effective contraception. There are clear medical grounds for termination of pregnancy in infected women.

### (f) Perinatal Transmission

Mother-to-infant HIV infection could be avoided if infected women would not become pregnant. Because of the potential high risk of infant infection and the preliminary clinical findings that pregnancy itself may accelerate the development of AIDS, it seems reasonable at this time to recommend that infected women postpone pregnancy.

## UNIVERSAL GENERAL PRECAUTIONS

The Centres for Disease Control has laid down certain recommendations that have to be used universally during all invasive procedures, in dentistry, dialysis, AIDS-laboratories and places where autopsy of AIDS patients is undertaken. Similar precautions have been *in vogue* while dealing with patients of viral hepatitis. Avoidance of contact with body secretions and blood of AIDS patient is very important because these are potentially infective. The likely situations of contact with the blood and body secretions include the sexual intercourse, kissing, handling the specimen of AIDS patients in laboratory, or during transfusion. These infected fluids should be carefully discarded after disinfection so as to prevent the accidental contamination. While dealing with these people, one should avoid chance wound. Similarly, the transport and subsequent autoclaving of the contaminated reusable items should be done very cautiously. Labelling of specimens should be a must, and appropriate warnings should be affixed.

**Table 12.1: Recommendations for Pathology Laboratories**

i) Avoid contact with skin and mucous membrane of blood or body secretions; use double gloves; wear goggles, mask and disposable waterproof gown; cover hair; minimize aerosolization of bone dust by using a vacuum attachment; prevent any abrasion or cut.

ii) Decontaminate instruments, containers, tissues and work area; decontaminate before discarding body fluids or contaminated water to sewage system.

iii) Identify and limit potential risk for others; Affix warning labels; do not distribute organs for transplantation or to random researchers; put cadavers in impervious bags.

iv) Limit access. Avoid pregnant, immunosuppressed or workers with abrasion/wounds; no other persons to be allowed in the laboratory.

The precautions recommended by the Laboratory of Pathology, National Cancer Institute, U.S.A, have been dealt with in Chapter 3. They deal with precautions during various histopathologic procedures (Table 12.1). Precautions should accordingly be taken when AIDS patients are investigated, or put on resuscitation unit. These instruments, such as bronchoscopes, sigmoidoscopes, respirators etc., should be placed in gluteraldeyde solutin immediately after the procedure, and kept at least for 30 minutes. They should then be washed and sterilised in ethylene dioxide before reusing.

## STERILIZATION AND DISINFECTION

Heat is the most effective method for inactivating HIV, thus autoclaving or boiling are the methods of choice. Chemical disinfectants are less reliable but useful in general laboratory decontamination. It is mandatory that all reusable instruments and equipments should be disinfected and cleaned thoroughly before they are preprocessed.

(i) Steam sterilization (Autoclaving) is the method or choice for reusable equipments, including needles and syringes. It is kept in operation for at least 20 minutes after a temperature of 121°c is reached.

(ii) Dry heat sterilization: Sterilization by dry heat is appropriate for instruments and equipments that can withstand a temperature of 170°C. Sterilization is accomplished at 160°C for a minimum of one hour.

(iii) Boiling: When an autoclave is not available, the simplest and most reliable method of inactivating most pathogenic microbes and HIV is by boiling. A high level of disinfection of instruments is achieved by continuous boiling for 20-30 minutes.

## CHEMICAL DISINFECTION

### 1. Chlorine-sodium hypochlorite

Sodium hypochlorite solution (liquid bleach) is an excellent universal disinfectant. A general all purpose laboratory disinfection solution for wiping work benches and specimens, containers, etc. is one with a concentration of 0.1% available chlorine (1 g/litre, 1000 ppm). A stronger solution for disinfecting heavily soiled equipment, blood spills etc. is one with a concentration of 1.0% available chlorine (10g/litre, 10000 ppm) Only fresh solutions should be used. The effectiveness of hypochlorite solution is reduced by blood, serum and other proteinacious material, so a regular replacement is required.

### 2. Chlorine-calcium hypochlorite

It decomposes at a slower rate than sodium hypochlorite and is formulated with 70% available chlorine. 0.1% solution is obtained by dissolving 1.4 g dry chemical in 1 litre of water. A 1.0% solution obtained by dissolving 14 g dry chemical in 1 litre of water.

### 3. Chloride sodium dischloroisocyanurate

It is normally formulated with 60% available chlorine in tablet form. At this strength, a 0.1% available chlorine solution is obtained by a dilution of 1.7 g stock in 1 litre of water. A 1.0% solution is obtained by dilution of 17 g stock in 1 litre of water. Tablets are also formulated at 1.5g of available chlorine per tablet. One tablet per litre of water provides a 0.1% solution for use. It is more stable than sodium and calcium hypochlorite.

### 4. Chloramine

It is normally formulated with 25% available chlorine. Because it releases chlorine at a slower rate than other chlorine compounds, higher concentrations are required for effective disinfection.

A dilution of 20 g stock in 1 litre of water is recommended as an all purpose disinfectant, while 40 g stock in 1 litre of water is recommended for disinfecting heavily soiled equipment, blood, spills etc. Chloramine is more stable than sodium and calcium hypochlorite.

### 5. Alcohol- ethanol (ethyl alcohol) and 2-propanol (isopropyl alcohol)

They are effective disinfectants, for wiping clean surfaces such as the exterior of specimen containers and bench tops. For the maximum effectiveness, they are used in a 70% concentration (70% alcohol, 30% water).

### 6. Iodophore- polyvidone iodine (PVI)

Iodophore disinfectant activity is similar to that of hypochlorite solution. Iodophores are more stable and less corrosive but expensive (do not use for aluminium or copper).

### 7. Formaldeyde- formalin

It is an excellent disinfectant, but its uses are limited because the solution and vapour released are toxic and very irritant. Formalin contains 35-40% formaldeyde, 10% methanol and water. It should be diluted 1:10

(a solution containing 3.5-4% formaldehyde) for disinfection. Rinse the equipment before reuse.

## 8. Gluteral-gluteraldeyde

Gluteraldehyde is a high level disinfectant, often used for the disinfection of non-disposable, heat-sensitive equipment and instruments. It is usually available as a 2% aqueous solution. To activate it, the powder or liquid supplied with the solution should be added.

Immersion in the solution destroys vegetative bacteria, fungi and viruses in less than 30 minutes. Ten hours immersion is required for the destruction of spores. Treated equipment must be thoroughly rinsed. Activated solutions should not be kept for over two weeks.

## ENVIRONMENTAL CONSIDERATIONS

Proper sterilization and disinfection of the reusable items, a satisfactory housekeeping when dealing with suspected infected material, cautious cleaning and decontamination of the spills of blood and body fluids, careful disposal of the infected waste and disposable items and an adequate laundry of the linen is mandatory keeping in view of environmental safety and prevention of transmission (Table 12.2).

## THE ROLE OF SEROLOGIC TESTING

The serologic test for HIV antibody is potentially an important tool for prevention.

### Infected Persons

If all infected (antibody-positive) individuals could be identified through voluntary and confidential testing programs and if these individuals could be counselled on ways to prevent exposure to others, then a major step toward decreasing AIDS could be achieved, Infected men and women could be advised of their risk to sexual partners or those exposed to their blood. Infected women could be advised to avoid pregnancy.

### Susceptible Persons

If uninfected (antibody-negative) individuals at increased risk of infection could be identified and counselled, their risk-taking behavior might decrease substantially.

In summary, serologic testing allows for knowledgeable clinical and preventive counselling of patients, including medical evaluation and

**Table 12.2: Prevention of AIDS**

1. Universal precautions to be taken in operation theatre, dentistry, autopsy, dialysis, and so on.
2. Avoid contact with blood/body secretions of AIDS and pre-AIDS.
3. Environmental considerations for sterilization and disinfection of contaminated reusable items and polluted work surfaces. Any spill of blood/ body fluid should be carefully cleaned.
4. Satisfactory house keeping while handling/transporting bags containing AIDS-related materials. Education courses should be given to members of housekeeping department.
5. Precaution to be observed in pathological laboratories; use disposable and impervious caps, goggles, gowns etc.
6. Proper labeling (PRECAUTION-AIDS/KS) of all AIDS-related materials, which should be placed in special plastic bags with zip.
7. Careful disposal of infected waste and disposable items after proper disinfection; avoid any accidental reuse.
8. In indoors, isolate the patient in single room but give him/her adequate moral courage.
9. Control of blood and blood-product is essential; donors should accordingly be screened; discourage unauthorised blood banks.
10. Avoid non-essential use of blood/blood products.
11. Plasma processing also requires certain prerequistes including reduction of number of donors contributing to a certain product; use specified donor material for a certain patient to prevent multiple donors exposures to him.
12. Precautions for health care personnel including those who have had exposures or have developed the disease.
13. Survillance of high-risk groups at fairly regular intervals.
14. HIV-1 testing for high-risk population, exposures, blood donors and suspected AIDS patient; and instructing them to observe precautions should they be positive for it.
15. Keep random researchers with inadequate facilities at bay.
16. Mass health education of the populations by the media such as newspapers, radio and television, highlighting means of prevention under different headings, like:
    - Avoid sex outside marriage
    - Avoid numerous sex partners
    - Avoid homosexual practices
    - Avoid drug abuse, and so on.

early intervention, personal counselling regarding decreasing transmission, contact tracing/notification, and counselling to prevent perinatal transmission.

## THE ROLE OF CONTACT TRACING/NOTIFICATION

The purpose of tracing sexual or needle-sharing contacts of infected people is to trace the chain of transmission to its terminus. At that point, there may be an infected person having risk-provoking contact with another susceptible person or persons. With appropriate education and motivation of the infected and susceptible contacts, further transmission can be prevented.

### Counselling

HIV/AIDS counselling is a relationship between patient and the counsellor with the aims of preventing transmission of HIV infection and providing psychosocial support to those already affected. It also provides support to the families of the infected people. Counselling seeks to help infected people make decisions about their life, boost their self confidence, improve relationship and quality of life. It can be provided apart from health care related setting, in any place where could be discussion about HIV or AIDS. Counsellors need not be formal health care providers; other motivated people can also provide counselling.

For people with HIV infection, individual and social adjustment involves lifelong stress management and adaptation. A broad range of physical problems which are not constant are likely to be experienced and these impose a variety of psychological and emotional stresses. Economic productivity may be affected and the direct and indirect financial costs imposed can be particularly telling. For the members of society at risk, counselling is essentially educative, with a knowledge of all aspects of the infection, providing the necessary impetus for behaviour change with a view of protecting themselves from acquiring the infection.

Counselling has to be an integral part of an HIV testing or screening programme. Prior to testing, the individual should be aware of the issues involved in testing and be sufficiently prepared for a positive test result. If tested negative, this pretest counselling would still form the basis for preventive inputs to maintain the noninfected status. If the infected person detected through testing, apart from the educative aspect with the emphasis on prevention of further spread from him, supportive aspects also gain prominence. This involves supporting the person from the shattering experience of the potentially terminal illness. Anticipation of possible reactions to the news of being infected and crisis situations likely to crop up and knowledge of strategies to tackle these are essential. It is also necessary for the family and friends of those infected and for the health care worker likely to come into contact with people with HIV infection of AIDS.

## NATIONAL AIDS CONTROL PROGRAMME PHASE-II (1999-2004)

The Phase II of the National AIDS Control Programme has become effective from 9th November, 1999. It is a 100% Centrally sponsored scheme implemented in 32 States/UTs and 3 Municipal Corporations namely Ahmedabad, Chennai and Mumbai through AIDS Control Societies. The three new states of Chattisgarh, Uttaranchal and Jharkhand are in the process of establishing their State AIDS Control Societies. It has two key objectives namely (a) to reduce the spread of HIV infection in India and (b) to strengthen the India's capability to respond to HIV/AIDS on a long term basis.

The programme has the following important targets to be achieved during project period:

(i) To reduce blood-borne transmission of HIV to less than one per cent of the total transmissions.

(ii) To introduce Hepatitis C as the fifth mandatory test for blood screening.

(iii) To set up 10 new modern blood banks in uncovered areas, upgrading of 20 major blood banks, setting up of 80 new district level blood banks in uncovered districts, establishing another 40 blood component separation units, promotion of voluntary blood donation and increase its share in total blood collected to at least 60%. The total blood collection in the country which is now around 3-3.5 million units is sought to be raised to 5-5.5 million units by the end of the project.

(iv) To attain awareness level of not less than 90% among the youth and those in the reproductive age group.

(v) To train at least 600 NGOs in the country in conducting targeted intervention programmes among high-risk groups and through them promote condom use of not less than 90% among these groups and control of STDs.

(vi) To conduct annual Family Health Awareness Campaigns among the general population and provide service-delivery in terms of medical advice and provision of drugs for control of STDs and Reproductive Tract Infections (RTIs). These campaigns will be conducted jointly by NACO and RHC programme managers at the State level.

(vii) Promotion of voluntary testing facilities across the country at the end of the project. It is visualised that every district in the country would have at least one voluntary testing facility.

(viii) Awareness campaigns will now be more interactive and use of traditional media such as folk arts and street theatre will be given greater priority in the rural areas. It is proposed to cover all the schools in the country targeting students studying in Class IX and Class XI through school education programmes and all the universities through the "Universities Talk AIDS" programme during the project period.

(ix) Promotion of Organisations of people living with HIV/AIDS and giving them financial support to form self-help groups.

NACO is leaving no stone unturned to uproot the AIDS menace from our country. It is targeting every possible route to control and eradicate HIV infection, viz.

1. Political advocacy
2. Blood Safety
3. Information, education, communication and social mobilization
4. Targetted interventions
5. Control of STDs and condom promotion
6. Family health awareness campaign
7. Prevention of mother to child transmission of HIV.
8. Prevention of AIDS in Health care workers and post-exposure prophylaxis.

   (For full details visit http://naco.nic.in/vsnaco/indianscene/country. htm)

# 13

# Afterthought

The emergence of AIDS has jolted the world. One of the way to combat this almost incurable disease has been to saturate the mass media with information packages containing probable cause of the disease, its nosology and symptomatology, and the precautions that are to be taken to avoid its infection. Several pragmatic as well as not-so-pragmatic suggestion have also been voiced to save the people form being gripped by this disease. The mass media have conscientiously warned the people that decline in human values, the sullying of moral standards, resorting to unnatural sexual practices, and turning against the well laid-out principles of nature can have disastrous consequences. A television programme on the decaying and dying AIDS patients is not only shuddering, but also convinces how dreadful the disease is, and such programmes are imperative in light of thousands of registered AIDS patients and the carriers of its virus, who are painfully waiting for their final departure.

Man-the Wise, as Oscar Wilde defined the taxonomic name *Homo sapiens,* has always tried demystify the mysteries of nature. He has devised means to harness the natural forces and use them for his survival. He has been chiefly concerned with 'mastering' the natural phenomena. In this process of gaining control over the nature, man has dishonoured the traditional yet commanding direction; the innate desire of man to domesticate the entire planet has unleashed a string of hitherto known terrors ranging from ecological degradation to the discovery of weapons that can potentially wipe out all the varieties of life from this world.

From such imbalances in nature have resulted those diseases which probably were confined to some remote species of animals. And perhaps these imbalances have yielded a sequel of certain complicated mutations in the existing group of viruses. An example of these processes of natural imbalances and mutations is AIDS. Introspecting the factors responsible for the advent, onslaught, and spread of this disease, we find that a majority of its patients are those who engaged themselves in homosexual acts-the acts which are unconceived and non-legitimized by nature. For nature, the pivotal aim of sexual union is procreation, and to this subjugated the pleasure principle. And once the pleasure principle overtakes the task of procreating one's own species, and when sex is treated intrinsically for detumescence, for pleasure *per se,* totally dissociated from moral concerns and a knowledge of proper natural laws, all kinds of perverted sex, an example of which is anal, start coming up. What the nature has regarded as base, fallen, and tabooed, is coming to occupy 'respectable' status in the Western world: there are widely publicized voluntary associations of gays and lesbians.

Once the homosexuals engage in heterosexual intercourses, they, quite unknowingly, spread the AIDS virus to their innocent female partners, who fall prey to the disease, and if they conceive, they usher in this world another innocent life caught by the macabre claws of this dreaded dragon. Similarly, the intra-venous drug abusers, unknown in what the anthropologists call the 'primitive' world, also suffer for their deeds by becoming another set of AIDS victims. Drug abuse has never been the 'survival need' of any organism, including man. We have discovered all these intoxicants by synthesizing the natural products, and for which were are paying through our nose. In addition to these, the patients who have to receive blood and blood product transfusion become unfortunate and chance victims of AIDS, if these components belong to the 'silent' AIDS patients. Fomites, of course, pay a role in transmitting AIDS, as they have been associated with the transmission of several infectious disorders since ages.

The relationship of AIDS with Western consummerism cannot be ruled out. The obsession to consume, and to treat every happiness as germinating from consumer patterns, including sex, has led to an exponential rise in moral chaos and disorders. Therefore, it is not astonishing that the panaceas the West suggests for saving oneself from the clutches of AIDS are masturbation, scourging the genitals and stimulating the lower parts of the body of one's partner, use of condoms, or what may be summed up in the term 'safe sex'. An Indian student studying in the West is taken aback when he receives a gift of condoms along with a plethora of literature on AIDS, or when he is advised to resort to masturbation, a habit he perhaps gave up in his adolescent years. It is indeed disheartening that in the list of panaceas for fighting AIDS, there is no mention, what to talk of emphasis, of monogamous sex or abstinence from it.

It is, therefore, high time that we endeavour to regain our moral standards and elevate ourselves in all facets of physical, mental, and spiritual vigour. It is high time that we condemn homosexuality, which is not only antithetical to natural laws, but also defies the thesis that males and females are complements in the same whole. It is high time that we inculcate these healthy moral values in our younger generation, exposing the noxious practices of homosexuality and drug abuse.

# Appendices

## Appendix I

Acquired Immunodeficiency Syndrome and HIV infection worldwide (Ref. world Health Organisation: Weekly Epidemiological Record 1999; 74: 401-408)

Reported AIDS cases as of November 15, 1999

| | |
|---|---|
| Africa | 794,444 |
| Americas | 1,010,193 |
| Eastern Mediterranean | 7917 |
| South-Asia | 140,246 |
| Europe | 224,404 |
| Western Pacific | 24,257 |
| Total | 2,201,461 |

**Africa**

| | |
|---|---|
| Algeria | 410 |
| Angola | 2433 |
| Benin | 2813 |
| Botswana | 10,142 |
| Burkina Faso | 13,518 |
| Burundi | 12,014 |
| Cameroon | 18,986 |
| Cape Verde | 269 |
| Central African Republic | 7016 |
| Chad | 10,121 |
| Comoros | 20 |
| Congo | 10,223 |
| Democratic Republic of the Congo | 47,557 |
| Ivory Coast | 49,532 |
| Equatorial Guinea | 321 |
| Eritrea | 6873 |
| Ethiopia | 37,874 |

**Africa**

| | |
|---|---|
| Rwanda | 15,903 |
| Sao Tome and Principe | 70 |
| Senegal | 2688 |
| Seychelles | 32 |
| Sierra Leone | 317 |
| South Africa | 12,825 |
| Swaziland | 3528 |
| United Republic of Tanzania | 112,052 |
| Togo | 10,827 |

| | |
|---|---|
| Uganda | 54,712 |
| Zambia | 44,942 |
| Zimbabwe | 74,782 |
| **Americas** | |
| Anguilla | 5 |
| Antigua and Barbuda | 96 |
| Antilles and Aruba | 257 |
| Argentina | 15,166 |
| Bahamas | 3098 |
| Barbados | 1043 |
| Belize | 198 |
| Bermuda | 346 |
| Bolivia | 179 |
| Brazil | 145,327 |
| British Virgin Islands | 16 |
| Gobon | 1660 |
| Gambia | 637 |
| Ghana | 29,546 |
| Guinea | 5307 |
| Guinea-Bissau | 823 |
| Kenya | 81,492 |
| Lesotha | 7317 |
| Liberia | 272 |
| Madagascar | 37 |
| Malawi | 50,975 |
| Mali | 5263 |
| Mauritania | 532 |
| Mauritius | 50 |
| Mozambique | 10,863 |
| Namibia | 6784 |
| Niger | 3644 |
| Nigeria | 26,276 |
| Reunion | 166 |
| Montserrat | 8 |
| Nicaragua | 182 |
| Panama | 1942 |
| Paraguay | 424 |
| Peru | 8940 |
| Saint Kitts and Nevis | 58 |
| Saint Lucia | 111 |
| Saint Vincent and the Grenadines | 139 |
| Suriname | 211 |
| Trinidad and Tobago | 2613 |
| Turks and Caicos Islands | 39 |
| United States | 717,430 |
| Uruguay | 1193 |
| Venezuela | 7282 |
| **Eastern Mediterranean** | |
| Afghanistan | – |
| Bahrian | 70 |
| Cyprus | 97 |
| Djibouti | 1783 |
| Egypt | 215 |
| Iran | 215 |
| Iraq | 108 |
| Jordan | 71 |
| Kuwait | 46 |
| Lebanon | 147 |
| Libyan Arab Jamahiriya | 32 |
| Morocco | 557 |
| Oman | 367 |
| Pakistan | 173 |
| Qatar | 93 |
| Saudi Arabia | 414 |
| Somalia | 13 |
| Sudan | 2735 |
| Syrian Arab Republic | 65 |
| Tunisia | 519 |
| United Arab Emirates | 8 |
| West Bank and Gaza Strip | 33 |
| Yemen | 156 |
| **Europe** | |
| Albania | 11 |
| Austria | 1915 |
| Armenia | 15 |
| Azerbaijan | 12 |
| Canada | 15,935 |
| Cayman Inlands | 24 |
| Chile | 2821 |
| Colombia | 8433 |
| Costa Rica | 1580 |
| Cuba | 864 |
| Dominica | 87 |
| Dominican Republic | 4733 |
| Ecuador | 872 |
| El Salvador | 2378 |
| French Guiana | 641 |
| Grenada | 103 |
| Guadeloupe | 790 |
| Guyana | 1053 |

| | |
|---|---|
| Haiti | 8899 |
| Honduras | 8217 |
| Jamaica | 2975 |
| Martinique | 436 |
| Mexico | 39,675 |
| **Europe** | |
| Belarus | 23 |
| Belgium | 2599 |
| Bulgaria | 60 |
| Bosnia and Harzagovina | 17 |
| Croatia | 144 |
| Czech Republic | 125 |
| Denmark | 2216 |
| Estonia | 22 |
| Finland | 294 |
| France | 49,421 |
| Georgia | 27 |
| Germany | 18,239 |
| Greece | 1964 |
| Hungary | 328 |
| Iceland | 50 |
| Ireland | 674 |
| Israel | 548 |
| Italy | 44,516 |
| Kyrgyzstan | 27 |
| Latvia | 37 |
| Lithuania | 26 |
| Luxembourg | 139 |
| Malta | 47 |
| Monaco | 40 |
| The Netherlands | 5054 |
| Norway | 638 |
| Poland | 794 |
| Portugal | 6020 |
| Republic of Moldova | 23 |
| Romaina | 5928 |
| Russian Federation | 395 |
| San Marino | 14 |
| Slovakia | 22 |
| Slovenia | 81 |
| Spain | 54,964 |
| Sweden | 1663 |
| Switzerland | 6641 |
| The Former Yugoslav Republic of Macedonia | 29 |
| Ukarine | 1022 |
| United Kingdom | 16,437 |
| Uzbekistan | 7 |
| Yugoslavia | 806 |
| **Southeast Asia** | |
| Bangladesh | 10 |
| Bhutan | – |
| Democratic Republic of Korea | – |
| India | 8438 |
| Indonexia | 265 |
| Maldives | 5 |
| Myanmar | 2568 |
| Nepal | 261 |
| Sri Lanka | 93 |
| Thailand | 128,606 |
| **Western Pacific** | |
| American Samoa | – |
| Australia | 8140 |
| Brunei Darussalam | 12 |
| Cambodia | 4834 |
| China | 419 |
| Cook Islands | – |
| Fiji | 8 |
| French Polynesia | 54 |
| Guam | 60 |
| Hong Kong Special Administrative Region of China | 409 |
| Japan | 2066 |
| Republic of Korea | 147 |
| Kiribati | 6 |
| Lao People's Democratic Republic | 105 |
| Macao | 17 |
| Malaysia | 2894 |
| Mariana Islands | 8 |
| Marshall Islands | 2 |
| Micronesia (Federated States of) | 2 |
| Mongolia | 1 |
| Nauru | – |

| | |
|---|---|
| New Caledonia and Dependencies | 67 |
| New Zealand | 681 |
| Niue | – |
| Palau | 1 |
| Papua New Guinea | 618 |
| Philippines | 404 |
| Samoa | 6 |
| Singapore | 545 |
| Solomon Islands | – |
| Tokelau | – |
| Tonga | 14 |
| Tuvalu | – |
| Vauatu | – |
| Vietnam | 2736 |
| Wallis and Futuna Islands | 1 |

Estimates of HIV/AIDS, 2003

| Region | Adults and Children Living with HIV/AIDS | Adults and Children Newly Affected with HIV during 2003 | Adult Prevalence (%)* | Adult and Child Deaths due to HIV/AIDS during 2003 |
|---|---|---|---|---|
| Sub-Saharan Africa | 25.0-28.2 million | 3.0-3.4 million | 7.5-8.5 | 2.2-2.4 million |
| North Africa and Middle East | 470,000-730,000 | 43,000-67,000 | 0.2-0.4 | 35,000-50,000 |
| South and Southeast Asia | 4.6-8.2 million | 610,000-1.1 million | 0.4-0.8 | 330,000-590,000 |
| East Asia and Pacific | 700,000-1.3 million | 150,000-270,000 | 0.1-0.1 | 32,000-58,000 |
| Latin America | 1.3-1.9 million | 120,000-180,000 | 0.5-0.7 | 49,000-70,000 |
| Caribbean | 350,000-590,000 | 45,000-80,000 | 1.9.3.1 | 30,000-50,000 |
| Eastern Europe and Central Asia | 1.2-1.8 million | 180,000-280,000 | 0.5-0.9 | 23,000-37,000 |
| Western Europe | 520,000-680,000 | 30,000-40,000 | 0.3-0.3 | 2,600-3,400 |
| North America | 790,000-1.2 million | 36,000-54,000 | 0.5-0.7 | 12,000-18,000 |
| Australia and New Zealand | 12,000-18,000 | 700-1000 | 0.1-0.1 | <100 |
| Total | 40 million (34-46 million) | 5 million (4.2-5.8 million) | 1.10% (0.9-1.3%) | 3 million (2.5-3.5 million) |

* The proportion of adults (15-49 years of age) living with HIV/AIDS in 2003, using 2003 population numbers.
(Data from AIDS Epidemic Update, Joint United Nations Programme on HIV/AIDS [UNAIDS] World Health Organization [WHO], December, 2003)

# Appendix II

Well-maintained data on incidence rates of AIDS in the United States (for case reported from July 1998 till June 1999).

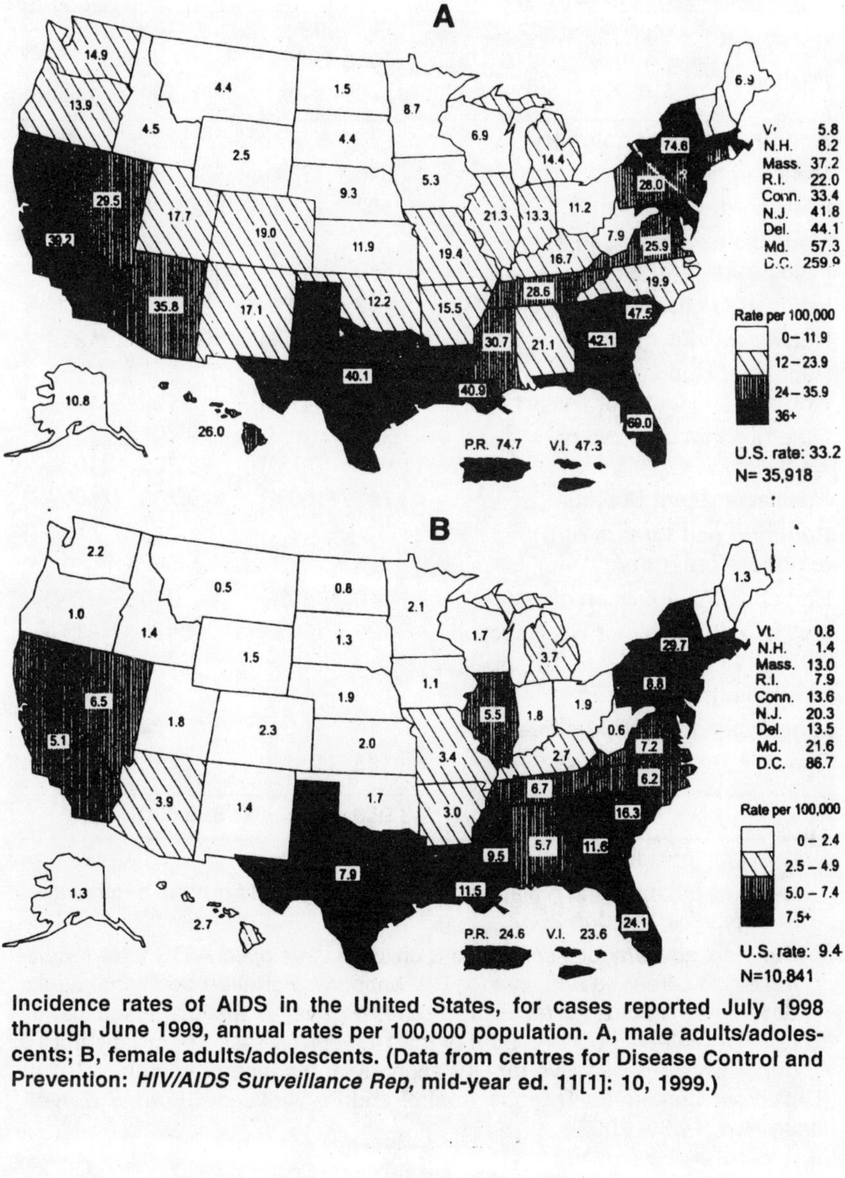


**Incidence rates of AIDS in the United States, for cases reported July 1998 through June 1999, annual rates per 100,000 population. A, male adults/adolescents; B, female adults/adolescents. (Data from centres for Disease Control and Prevention: *HIV/AIDS Surveillance Rep,* mid-year ed. 11[1]: 10, 1999.)**

# Appendix III

AIDS Cases by Age Group and Exposure Category, Through December 2002 and Cumulative Totals Through December 2002, United States

| | July 1998 to June 1999 | | Cumulative Total* | |
|---|---|---|---|---|
| | No. | (%) | No. | (%) |
| **Adult/adolescent category** | | | | |
| Men who have sex with men | 14,545 | (33%) | 384,784 | (45%) |
| Injecting drug use | 7502 | (17%) | 209,920 | (25%) |
| Men who have sex with men and inject drugs | 1510 | (3%) | 54,224 | (6%) |
| Hemophilia/coagulation disorder | 90 | (0%) | 5371 | (1%) |
| Heterosexual contact | 7953 | (16%) | 100,071 | (12%) |
| Receipt of blood transfusion, blood components, or tissue† | 265 | (1%) | 9152 | (1%) |
| Other/risk not reported or identified | 11,927 | (27%) | 86,258 | (10%) |
| Adult/adolescent Subtotal | 43,792 | (100%) | 849,780 | (100%) |
| **Pediatric (< 13 years old) exposure category** | | | | |
| Hemophilia/coagulation disorder | 0 | (0%) | 236 | (3%) |
| Mother with/at risk for HIV infection | 139 | (88%) | 8425 | (91%) |
| Receipt of blood transfusion, blood components, or tissue† | 2 | (1%) | 385 | (4%) |
| Other/risk not reported or identified | 17 | (11%) | 174 | (2%) |
| Pediatric Subtotal | 158 | (100%) | 9220 | (100%) |
| Total | 43,950 | | 859,000 | |

**Note:** Total includes 2 persons whose sex is unknown.

* Includes persons with a diagnosis of AIDS, reported from the beginning of the epidemic through 2002.

† Forty-six adults/adolescents and 3 children developed AIDS after receiving blood screened negative for HIV antibody. Fourteen additional adults developed AIDS after receiving tissue, organs, or artificial insemination from HIV-infected donors. Four of the 14 received tissue or organs from a donor who was negative for HIV antibody at the time of donation.

(Data from Centers for Disease Control and Prevention: *HIV/AIDS Surveillance Rep,* 14:30, 2002.)

# Appendix IV

## QUESTIONS – YOUNG MEN AND WOMEN ASK THE DOCTOR REGARDING AIDS AND OTHER SEXUALLY TRANSMITTED DISEASES

Q.1. What is a venereal disease?

A.1 Venereal diseases are a group of diseases that are infective in origin and transmitted through sexual intercourse and intimate love making. They are also called sexually-transmitted diseases (STDs).

Q.2. How do they occur?

A.2. They occur primarily in, and also transmitted through, those persons who do not observe strict marital sex. They are promiscuous and indulge in frequent sex with numerous sexual partners. These diseases don't occur in normal married couples who don't keep extramarital affairs.

Q.3. How do they present?

A.3. They present with either bruises, painful/painless ulcers and growths, or with discharge through urinary tract and/or vagina, following a variable period after sexual intercourse with an infected male/female.

Q.4. Name some important venereal diseases?

A.4. Common venereal diseases presenting with sore on the genitalia are syphilis, chancroid, herpes, donovanosis & lymphogranuloma venereum; those presenting with overgrowth include genital warts and molluscum, while purulent discharge through genital orifices is seen in gonococcal infections, trichomoniasis and candidiasis.

Q.5. What is HIV?

A.5. HIV (human immunodeficiency virus) is the virus that causes AIDS. This virus is transmitted through blood-to-blood and sexual contact. In addition, infected pregnant women can pass HIV to their baby during pregnancy or delivery, as well as through breast-feeding. People with HIV have HIV infection, most of them will develop AIDS.

Q.6. Is AIDS also a venereal disease?

A.6. AIDS is also a venereal disease, as majority of its victims are homosexual males, and their heterosexual female partners. However, it can be transmitted through non-venereal means also, such as people who inject themselves with infected needles, through blood transfusions and so on.

Q.7. Where did HIV come from?

A.7. Scientists have different theories about the origin of HIV, but none have been proven. The earliest known case of HIV was from a blood sample collected in 1959 from a man in Kinshasha, Democratic Republic of Congo. (How he became infected is not known.) Genetic analysis of this blood sample suggests that HIV-1 may have stemmed from a single virus in the late 1940s or early 1950s. The virus has existed in the United States since at least the mid-to late 1970s. From 1979-1981 rare types of pneumonia, cancer, and other illnesses were being reported by doctors in Los Angeles and New York among a number of gay male patients. They were usually not found in people with healthy immune systems. In 1982 public health officials began to use the term “acquired immunodeficiency syndrome”, or AIDS, to describe the occurrences of opportunistic infections, Kaposi’s sarcoma, and Pneumocystis carinii pneumonia in previously healthy men. Formal tracking (surveillance) of AIDS cases began that year in the United States.

Q.8. Who is a homosexual?

A.8. A homosexual is a person who indulges in sexual practices with partners of his own sex. They are usually males, and frequently have anal-intercourse. They can also have sexual relationships with people of opposite sex (heterosexual) and thus may transmit disease organisms from one person to other.

Q.9. Does AIDS also has the same presenting features?

A.9. AIDS has a bit complex presentation. Though, transmitted chiefly through sexual intercourse, it may not show the usual ulceration or discharge through the genitalia, but rather a life-threatening serious systemic and extensive disease i.e. severe infective illness or unusual cancers.

Q.10. By the way what is AIDS?

A.10. AIDS is an abbreviated form of *Acquired Immuno-Deficiency Syndrome.* It denotes an acquired deficiency and failure of the defensive system of the body. This defensive system of our body combats with any invading micro-organism and prevents its foot-hold in the body. It also kills certain abnormal cells that incidentally form amongst the dividing cells of our body. Thus, absence of this protective system will (i) allow the invading organisms to germinate in the body, disseminate, and cause widespread disease, (ii) allow the abnormal clones of cells to divide further, and thus produce cancers.

Q.11. How this failure of our defensive system occur?

A.11. This failure results from the widespread death of those cells of blood ($T_4$ type white blood cells) who regulate this defence, caused by the micro-organism of AIDS infection. The virus keeps on having strong foot-hold in the body of the victim and causing gradually complete collapse of the defence system. The further damage to the body is caused by other invading organisms to whose entry the body can not resist. Also, cancer cells start proliferating in the body.

Q.12. What are the suspicion arouser that a patient is afflicted with AIDS?

A.12. Fortunately, AIDS is predominently seen in certain groups of individuals who are at a high risk for its development. They are homosexual males, intravenous drug abusers, people who require repeated blood/blood product transfusion, haemophiliacs, sexual partners and children of AIDS patients, and people of certain geographic areas such as Haiti. Thus, first suspicion arouser is that the person belongs to one of these groups. The other suspicion arousers are the sudden excessive loss of weight, fever, and cough which do not respond to routine treatment for long periods, and other unusually prolonged diseases who don't resolve even after extensive treatment. Another suspicion arouser is the occurrence of cancers in young adult-hood.

Q.13. How do people get infected with HIV?

A.13. HIV is transmitted mostly through semen and vaginal fluids during unprotected sex. In some developed countries homosexual activity remains the primary mode. Besides sexual intercourse, HIV can also be transmitted during drug injection by the sharing of needles contaminated with infected blood; by the transfusion, of infected blood or blood products; and from an infected woman to her baby – before birth, during birth or just after delivery. HIV does not spread through ordinary social contact; for example by shaking hand, travelling in the same bus, eating from the same utensils, by hugging Mosquitoes and insects do not spread the virus nor is it water-borne or air-borne.

Q.14. How many people are infected with HIV?

A.14. According to UNAIDS estimates, by December-2003, nearly 34-46 million people including over 2.5 million children – had been infected with HIV since the Number of people living with HIV/AIDS Total 40 million (34 - 46 million)

- Adults 37 million (31 - 43 million)
- Children under 15 years 2.5 million (2.1 - 2.9 million)
- People newly infected with HIV in 2003 Total 5 million (4.2 - 5.8 million)
- 4.2 million (3.6 - 4.8 million)
- Children under 15 years 700 000 (590 000 - 810 000)
- AIDS deaths in 2003 Total 3 million (2.5 - 3.5 million)
- Adults 2.5 million (2.1 - 2.9 million)
- Children under 15 years 500 000 (420 000 - 580 000)

Q.15. Can any medicine or drug kill this AIDS-virus, or if any vaccination renders immunity against it?

A.15. Till date, no drug is discovered that can kill this virus inside human body. However, antiretroviral drugs given indefinitely can control viral replication. That is why it is yet regarded as an non-curable disease. So, every patient of AIDS will be presumed to die in a few months or years, depending upon the severity of infection, and/or fulminancy of the carcinomas they develop. At present, no effective vaccine has been developed for AIDS-virus, but in near future, the scientists working vigorously on this aspect, may develop an effective vaccine to immunize the susceptible population.

Q.16. I have indulged in pre/extra-marital contact. I am scared if I will develop AIDS?

A.16. AIDS can affect people if they have numerous sexual partners, people who are promiscuous. Fortunately, the cases of AIDS recorded in India are only sporadic, and thus the reservoirs of AIDS virus may also be few. But there are all the possibilities that sexual intercourse outside marriage may transmit AIDS to young healthy adults, especially if they are with unknown partners who have previously resided abroad or in areas where AIDS has been discovered.

Q.17. I have been a homosexual person, and occasionally indulge in such activities. I understand, homosexual men are the commonest AIDS victims. Please guide me?

A.17. No doubt, majority of AIDS patients have been homosexual men.

They are also offenders in spreading AIDS to their wives as well. But it is never too late. Please stop all homosexual contacts immediately. Keep yourself busy so that you do not get tempted towards your past habits. As told earlier, AIDS has not assumed alarming proportions in India, so it is unlikely that you might have contacted AIDS. However, you may be the prospective victim of AIDS in near future if you don't stop anal intercourse.

Q.18. I am a drug abuser, injecting with my syringe drugs in me and my friends time and again. Please advise.

A.18. Yes, you are another likely candidate to develop this dreaded disease. Infected needles easily spread AIDS. Stop this habit henceforth, otherwise you are heading two folds towards death one from these drugs, the other if you accidently get AIDS.

Q.19. I am suffering form certain disease which require repeated blood transfusions, which is equally important for my survival. Please enlighten me.

A.19. As you require repeated blood transfusions, please ensure that you go to hospitals/nursing homes where strict precautions are taken before transfusing blood, including testing the blood donors as well as stored blood for AIDS antibodies. Don't use unauthorised blood from other sources, who sell contaminated blood. Hospitals and nursing homes undertake utmost precautions in this regard. So, please do not bother if you are only getting transfusions in reliable medical centres.

Q.20. My husband is promiscuous. What should I do?

A.20. It is very difficult for ladies like you, but make efforts to dissuade your husband from having sex outside marriage. If accidentally he becomes HIV positive, he may ruin his whole family. You both should get blood tested for AIDS for early detection, and if tested negative, take strict precautions in future and practise safe sex.

Q.21. I am a HIV-positive housewife. I want to bear children. Is it safe?

A.21. It is very unsafe to bear children if you are HIV-positive, as chances are very high that you will infect your child in pregnancy, during delivery or during lactation with AIDS virus.

Q.22. How does a mother transmit HIV to her unborn child?

A.22. An HIV-infected mother can infect the child in her womb through her blood. The baby is more at risk if the mother has been recently infected or is in a later stage of AIDS. Transmission can also occur to the time of birth and to some extent transmission can occur through breast milk. Transmission from an infected mother to her baby occurs in about 30% of cases.

Q.23. Can HIV be transmitted through breast-feeding?

A.23. The virus has been found in breast milk in low concentrations and studies have shown that children of HIV-infected mothers can get HIV infection through breast milk. Breast milk, however, has many substances in it that protect an infant's health and the benefits of breast-feeding for both mother and child are well recognized. The slight risk of an infant becoming infected with HIV through breast-feeding is therefore thought to be outweighed by the benefits of breast-feeding.

Q.24. Is Oral Sex Unsafe?

A.24. Oral sex does carry some risk of infection. If a person sucks the penis of an infected man, for example, infected fluid could get into the mouth. The virus could then get into the blood if you have tiny sores somewhere in the mouth. The same is true if infected sexual fluids from a woman get into the mouth of her partner.

Q.25. Can I get HIV from getting a tattoo or through body piercing?

A.25. A risk of HIV transmission does exist if instruments contaminated with blood are used inappropriately between clients. CDC recommends that instruments that are intended to penetrated the skin be used once, then disposed of or thoroughly cleaned and sterilized. Personal service workers who do tattooing body piercing should be educated about how HIV is transmitted and take precautions to prevent transmission of HIV and other blood-borne infections in their settings.

Q.26. Can I get infected with HIV from mosquitoes?

A.26. From the start of the HIV epidemic there has been concern about HIV transmission of the virus by biting and bloodsucking insects, such as mosquitoes. However, studies conducted by the CDC and elsewhere have shown no evidence of HIV transmission through mosquitoes or any other insects – even in areas where there are many cases of AIDS and large populations of mosquitoes.

Q.27. I am a social worker dealing with terminally ill patients including AIDS. what precautions I should take?

A.27. AIDS is only transmitted through body secretions of the affected people. Take care not to let these infected materials to come in contact with any wound on your body while serving these hapless victims.

Q.28. I feel very sorry to see innocent victims of AIDS—infants and children. Can I help?

A.28. We all can help by creating awareness about AIDS in our country. By educating our people we can prevent promisquity and subsequent spread of the disease to pregnant mother. Should a female becomes HIV positive she should be encouraged to avoid pregnancy at all cost to prevent pediatric AIDS.

Q.29. What are rapid HIV tests?

A.29. A rapid test for detecting antibody to HIV is a screening test that produces very quick results, usually in 5 to 30 minutes. In comparison, results from the commonly used HIV antibody-screening test, the EIA (enzyme immunoassay), are not available for 1-2 weeks. Both the rapid test and the EIA look for the presence of antibodies to HIV. As is true for all screening tests (including the EIA), a reactive rapid HIV test result must be confirmed before a diagnosis of infection can be given.

Q.30. Are there other tests available?

A.30. The EIA (enzyme immunoassay) is the standard screening test used to detect the presence of antibodies to HIV. The EIA should be used with a confirmatory test such as the Western blot. Other tests now available include:

- Radioimmunoprecipitation assay (RIPA): A confirmatory blood test that may be used when antibody levels are very low or difficult to detect or when Western blot test results are uncertain. An expensive test, the RIPA requires time and expertise to perform.
- Rapid latex agglutination assay: A simplified, inexpensive blood test that may prove useful in medically disadvantaged areas where there is a high prevalence of HIV infection.
- Dot-blot immunobinding assay: A rapid-screening blood test that is cost-effective and that may become an alternative to conventional EIA and Western blot testing.
- Antigen capture assay: Also known as the HIV-1 antigen capture assay. The Food and Drug Administration (FDA) added this blood test as an interim measure in 1996 to HIV-antibody testing to protect the blood supply further until other tests become available to detect early HIV infection before antibodies are fully developed. Because some activity of p24 antigen is unpredictable, this test is not useful for helping people find out if they have HIV.
- Polymerase chain reaction (PCR): A specialized blood test that looks for HIV genetic information. Although expensive and

labor-intensive, the test can detect the virus even in someone only recently infected. To further protect the blood supply, the FDA has indicated that the development and implementation of tests of HIV genetic material such as PCR is warranted.

Q.31. Is there a vaccine for HIV/AIDS? What is WHO'S role is this regard?

A.31. While there is currently no vaccine for HIV/AIDS, research is under way many candidate vaccines are presently undergoing either phase I or phase II clinical trials in various countries, including Thailand in South-East Asia. These will be followed by field trials in the community to determine efficacy. Hence, a vaccine for general use is unlikely to be available in the near future. WHO's role is to assist in the development, evaluation and availability of vaccines. WHO has helped four countries – Brazil, Rwanda, Thailand and Uganda – to prepare a comprehensive plan for HIV vaccine research including strengthening of national epidemiological, laboratory and socio-behavioural research capabilities.

Q.32. Is there a treatment for HIV/AIDS?

A.32. All the currently licensed anti-retroviral drugs, namely AZT, ddl and ddC, have effects which last only for a limited duration. In addition, these drugs are very expensive and have severe adverse reactions while the virus tends to develop resistance rather quickly with single-drug therapy. The emphasis is now on giving a combination of drugs including newer drugs called protease inhibitors; but this makes treatment even more expensive. WHO's present policy advocates strengthening of clinical management for HIV-associated opportunistic infections such as tuberculosis and diarrhoea. Better care programmes have been shown to prolong survival and improve the quality of life of people living with HIV/AIDS.

Q.33. I understand that prevention of AIDS is the only solution. What precautions we people should take to keep ourselves safe?

A.33. A clear understanding of this disease, its various manifestations and routes of transmission, is the first and foremost preventive measure that will go a long way in controlling this disease. Observe high morals of sex, and have sex only within marriage. Avoid drug abuse. For getting infections or transfusions, use disposable syringes and needles. Other precautions have been summarised in Chapter 12.

# Appendix V

## SIGNIFICANCE OF A LABORATORY TEST

A. Specificity: Ratio of true negatives to the sum of false positive and true negatives i.e. III/II+III

B. Sensitivity: Ratio of true positives to the sum of true positives and false negatives i.e. I/I+IV

| Permutations to test | Presence of Disease | HIV-1 antibodies | Inference |
|---|---|---|---|
| I | + | + | True positive |
| II | – | + | False positive |
| III | – | – | True negative |
| IV | + | – | False negative |

C. Precision: It is the correlation of absorbance measured in duplicate tests.

D. Reproducibility: A test is called reproducible if the ratio of results on any single serum done on two separate occasions is one or very close to it.

# APPENDIX VI

## NACO: STATE AIDS CONTROL SOCIETIES

| S.No. | Project Director | Address |
|---|---|---|
| 01. | Dr. R. Thulasidasan | Andaman & Nicobar AIDS Control Society, G.B. Pant Hospital Complex, Port Blair-744104 |
| 02. | Smt. K Damayanthi, IAS | Andhra Pradesh State AIDS Control Society, Directorate of Medical & Health Services, Sultan Bazar, Hyderabad-500059 |
| 03. | Dr. Hage Lodar | Arunachal Pradesh Arunachal Pradesh AIDS Control Society, Naharlagun, New Itanagar-791110 |
| 04. | Shri J.C. Dewri | Assam State AIDS Control Society, Khanapara, Guwahati-781 022 |
| 05. | Sh. C.K. Anil, IAS | Bihar State AIDS Control Society, Health Department, New Secretariat, Patna-800 015 |
| 06. | Dr. N.M. Sharma | Chandigarh Chandigarh AIDS Control Society, SCO No. 14-15, 1st Floor, Sector 8-C, Chandigarh-160018 |
| 07. | Dr. L.N. Patra | Dadra & Nagar Haveli AIDS Control Society, I Floor, Shri Vinoda Bhave Civil Hospital, Silvassa-396230 |
| 08. | Dr. S.S. Vaishya | Daman & Diu AIDS Control Society, UT of Daman & Diu, Primary Health Centre, Moti Daman-396220 |
| 09. | Shri. Arun Baroka | Delhi B.S. Ambedkar Hospital, 1st and 2nd Floor, Dharamsala Block Rohini Sector-6, Delhi 10085 |
| 10. | Dr. P.K. Ghodge | Goa First Floor Dayanand Smiriti Building, Swami Vivekanand Road, Panaji-403001 |
| 11. | Dr. G.S. Rore | Gujarat State AIDS Control Society 0/1 Block, New Mental Hospital Complex, Menghaninagar, Ahmedabad-380016 |
| 12. | Sri. B.S. Dahiya | Haryana AIDS Control Society, SCO-10, Sector-10, Panchkula |

*(Contd.)*

| S.No. | Project Director | Address |
|---|---|---|
| 13. | Dr. R.N. Mahanta | Himachal Pradesh State AIDS Control Society, Block No. 38, Ground Floor, SDA Complex, Kasumpti, Shimla-171009 |
| 14. | Dr. M.A. Wani | J&K State AIDS Prevention Control Society, 1st Floor, Khyber Hotel, Khayam Chowk, Srinagar |
| 15. | Mrs. T. Mukthamba | Karnataka State AIDS Control Society, No. 4/13-1, Crescent Road, High Grds Bangalore-560001 |
| 16. | Dr. Rajan Khobragade, IAS | Kerala State AIDS Control Society, IPP Building, Red Cross Road, Thiruvanathapuram, Kerala-695037 |
| 17. | Dr. Atta Koya | Lakshadweep AIDS Control Society, Directorate of Medical & Health Services, UT of Lakshadweep, Kavaratti-682555 |
| 18. | Ms. Salina Singh | Madhya Pradesh AIDS Control Society, OILFED Building, 1 Arera Hills, Bhopal-462011 |
| 19. | Shri. Sanjay Sawant | Maharastra SACS, Ackworth Leprosy Hosp. Comp, Behind S.I.W.S. College, R.A. Kidwai Marg, Wadala (West), Mumbai-400031 |
| 20. | Dr. S. Sukumar Singh | Manipur SAC Society, Medical Directorate, R & D Wing, Lamphelpat, Imphal-795004 |
| 21. | Dr. P.K. Barooah | Meghalaya AIDS Control Society, Ideal Lodge, Oakland, Shillong-793001 |
| 22. | Dr. K. Ropari | Mizoram AIDS Control Society, MV-124, Mission Veng South, Aizawl-796005 |
| 23. | Dr. Kumuni Kathipri | Nagaland State AIDS Control Society, Medical Directorate, Kohima-797001 |
| 24. | Sri Mayadhar Panigrahi, IAS | Orissa State AIDS Control Society, Oil Orissa Building, Nayapalli, Bhubaneshwar |
| 25. | Dr. G Fernandez | Pondicherry AIDS Society No. 93, Perumal kail Street, Pondicherry |

*(Contd.)*

| S.No. | Project Director | Address |
|---|---|---|
| 26. | Mr. Sukhpal Singh Gill, IAS | Punjab State AIDS Control Society, SCO No. 481-82, Sector 35-C, Chandigarh |
| 27. | Dr. D. Mathur | Rajasthan State AIDS Control Society, Medical & Health Directorate, Swasthya Bhawan, Tilak Marg, "C" Scheme, Jaipur-302005 |
| 28. | Dr. R.L. Sharma | Sikkim State AIDS Control Society, STNM Hospital, Gangtok-737101 |
| 29. | Shri. S. Vijay Kumar | Tamil Nadu State AIDS Control Society, 417, Pantheon Road, Egmore, Chennai-600008 |
| 30. | Dr. Tapan Kumar Das | Tripura SAC Society, Health Directorate Building, Gurkhabasti, P.O. Kunjaban, Agartala, West Tripura-799006 |
| 31. | Ms. C.B. Paliwal, IAS | U.P. State AIDS Control Society, 'A' Block, 4th Floor, PICUP Bhawan, Gomti Nagar, Lucknow-226010 |
| 32. | Sh. S.Suresh Kumar, IAS | West Bengal SACS, Swastha Bhavan, GN-29, Sector V, Salt Lake Kolkata-700091 |
| 33. | Dr. Laxman Melodia | Ahmedabad MC Society, Old Municipal Dispensary, Behind Lal Bungalow, C.G. Road, Ahmedabad. |
| 34. | Mr. Sundara Murthy, IAS | Chennai Municipal Corporation AIDS Prevention & Control Society, 82 Thiru Vi-Ka Salai, Mylapore Chennai-600003 |
| 35. | Dr. Alka Gogate | Mumbai District AIDS Control Society, Hospital Compound, Behind S.I.W.S. College, R.A. Kidwai Marg, Wadala (West), Mumbai-31 |
| 36. | Shri. Rajiv Arun Ekka, IAS | Jharkhand AIDS Control Society, Sadar Hosp. Camp. Purulia Road, |
| 37. | Dr. G.S. Jangpangi | Uttaranchal State AIDS Control Society, Chandar Nagar, Dehradun |
| 38. | Dr. S.K. Kehri | Chattisgarh AIDS Control Society, Directorate of Health Services, State Health Training Centre, Near Kalibadi Chowk, Raipur |

# Appendix VII

## CAN THIS BE AIDS?

Acquired immunodeficiency syndrome does not show its own characteristics *per se,* rather it expresses itself in diverse and confusing ways. Nevertheless, such bizarre presentations do give an inkling about this underlying horror. Its cutaneous indicators are sometimes extensive and horrible, but may often be trivial, yet persistent and recurrent. However, all extensive dermatoses may not be dangerous as AIDS, and all trivial manifestations may not be inocuous in AIDS patient. The following photographs highlight the preceding fact, and some are a few examples of an infinite spectrum of AIDS.

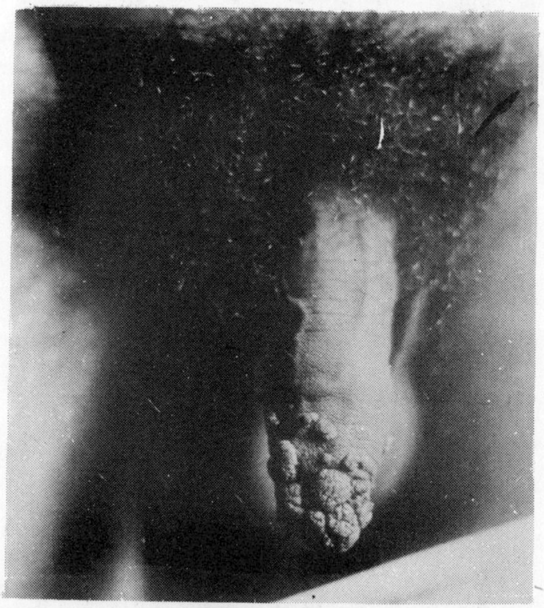

**Fig. 1. Genital warts on the penis. The occurrence of genital warts, although not a regular AIDS feature, often signifies the promiscuous status of the patients, as it is a sexually transmitted disease. People with multiple sexual partners, and consequently with repeated history of sexually-transmitted diseases are more likely to get an exposure to AIDS virus.**

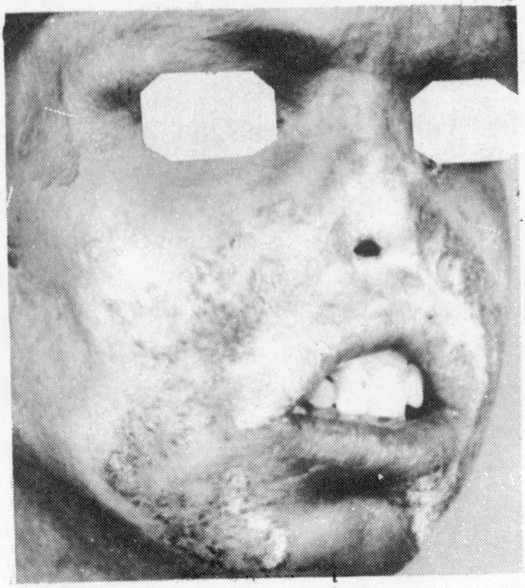

**Fig. 2. Lupus vulgaris on face causing disfiguration. (Courtesy Sehgal et al, Clinical and Experimental Dermatology, 1988). This variety of skin tuberculosis occurs in persons with a relatively strong immunity to *M. tuberculosis.* Although tuberculosis is now increasingly seen in AIDS patients, yet this variety is unlikely to be seen in AIDS.**

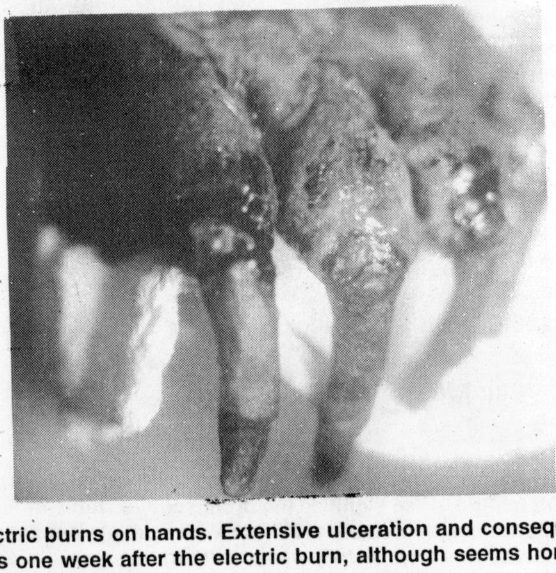

**Fig. 3. Electric burns on hands. Extensive ulceration and consequent necrosis of the digits one week after the electric burn, although seems horrible, yet has nothing to do with AIDS.**

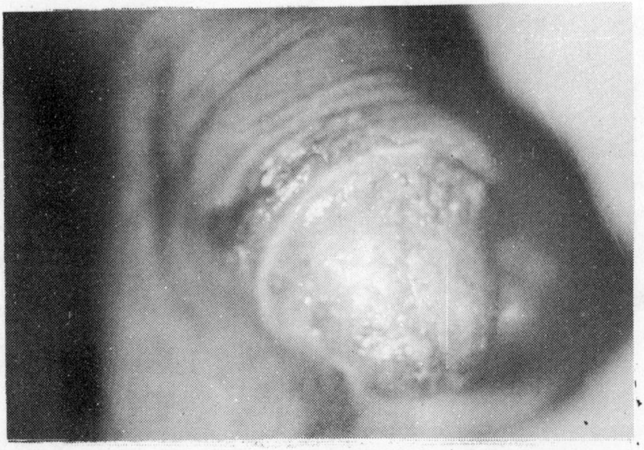

Fig. 4. Fixed drug eruption on glans penis. This peculiar drug eruption has a prediliction for glans penis, and presents as painful dusky red localized erosion. Its sudden occurrence after ingestion of sulfa or pain-relieving drugs surprises the patient. AIDS patients, however, may fail to reveal drug eruptions!

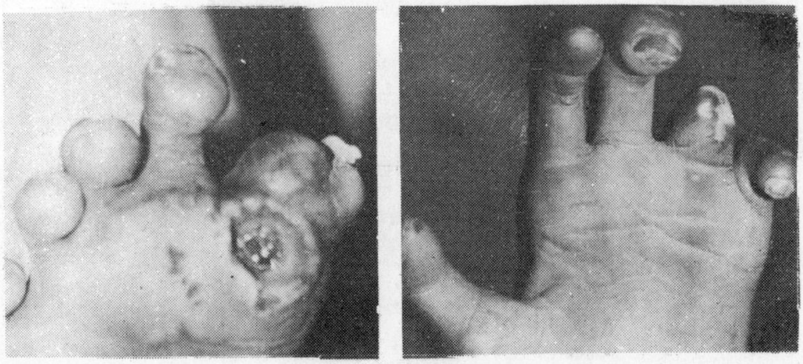

**Fig. 5. (a) & (b) Deformity, ulcerations and absorption of toes and fingers consequent to loss of sensations in leprosy. Leprosy is fairly common in India and often cause deformities and disabilities. AIDS and leprosy may coexist and the latter may became florid due to immunodepression caused by AIDS.**

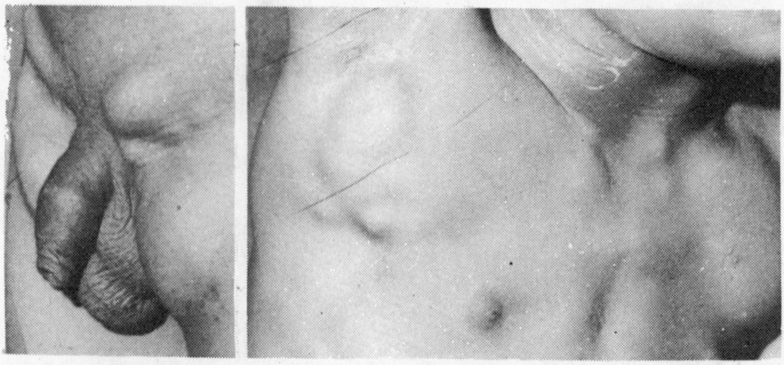

**Fig. 6. (a) & (b) Lymphoplastic lymphoma with leukaemia. Note the extensive lymphadenopathy in the axillae and groin. The persistent generalized lymphadenopathy of AIDS usually does not ever attain this big size. However lymphomas can supervene on AIDS.**

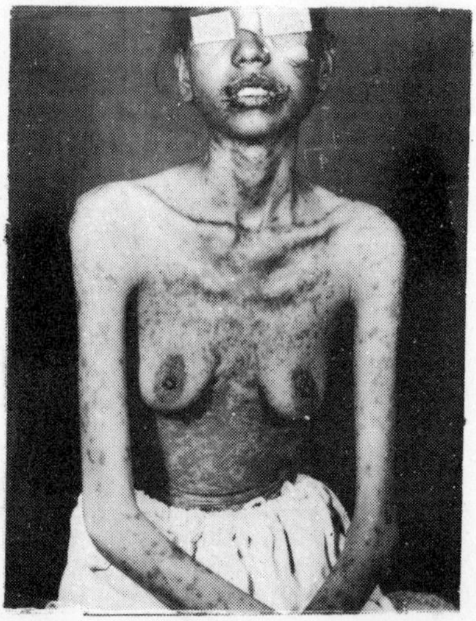

**Fig. 7. Stevens Johnson syndrome in a young female of 21 years suffering from pulmonary tuberculosis. It can be induced by several drugs including anti-tubercular medicines. It is a severe from of erythema multiformae. Adverse reactions to drugs can also be seen in AIDS and are of serious import.**

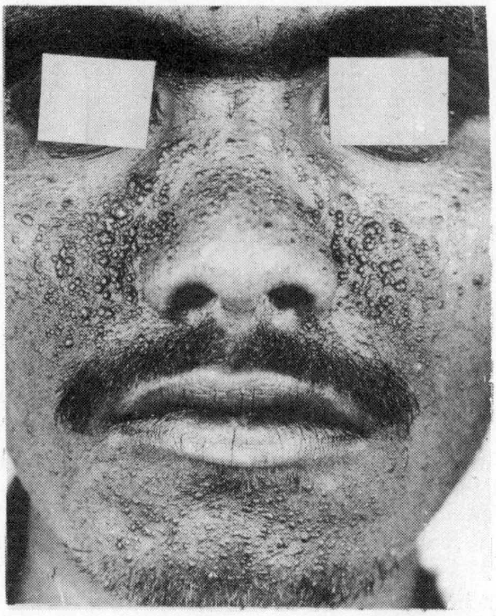

**Fig. 8. Adenoma sebaceum. This benign tumour of young adults is cosmetically embarassing. Some times it is associated with epilepsy. It has nothing to do with AIDS.**

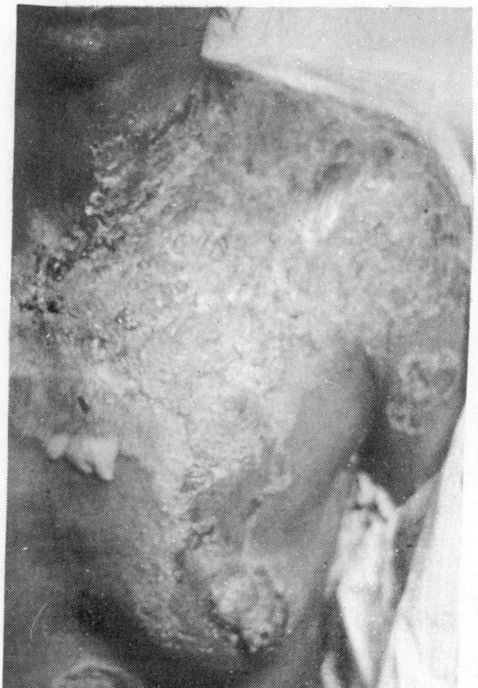

**Fig. 9. Pemphigus vulgaris, a chronic vesicobullous autoimmune disorder can affect both sexes. Running a prolonged course of exacerbation and remitting with cortico-steroid treatment, it rather requires immuno-suppressants for control. AIDS may cause it remit!**

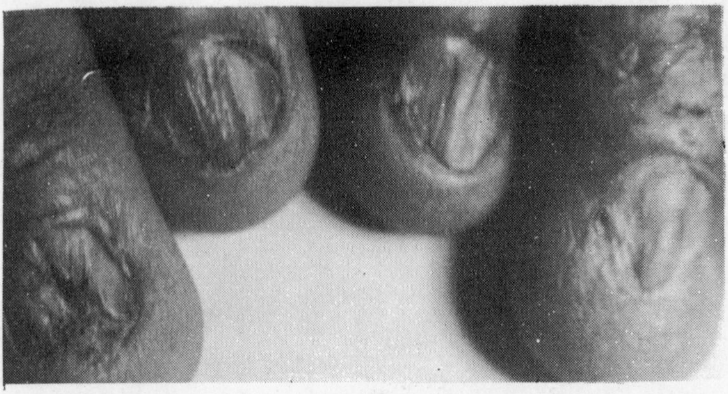

Fig. 10. Nail dystrophy induced by lichen planus. All twenty nails may show signs of damage. Its exact etiology is not known. Yellow nail syndrome of nails in AIDS is usually seen to result from chronic pulmonary infections.

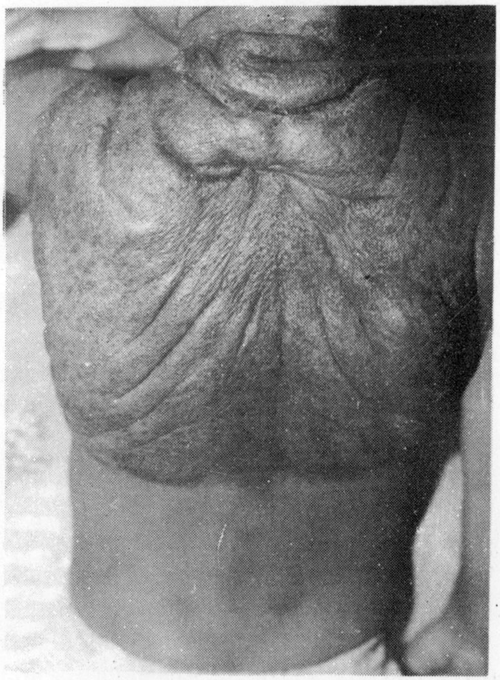

Fig. 11. Giant congenital pigmented nevus with features of plexiform neurofibromatosis. A congenital disorder, sometime associated with other developmental abnormalities, is definitely less repulsive than AIDS.

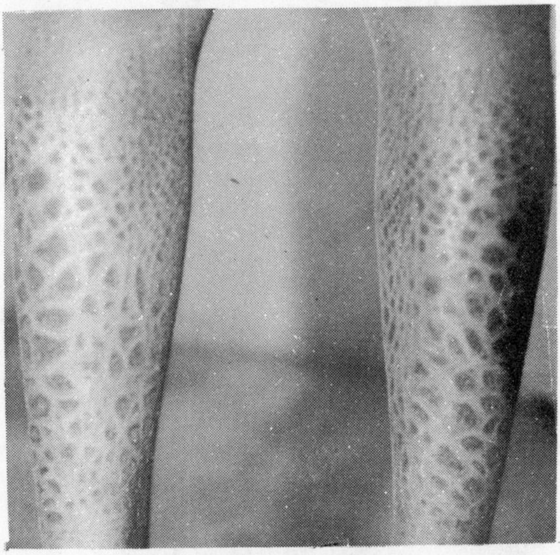

**Fig. 12. X-linked, ichthyosis, a hereditary xerotic skin disorder. Xeroderma simulating ichthyosiform dermatitis can be seen in pediatric AIDS, chiefly due to nutritional deficiency and incidious wasting illness.**

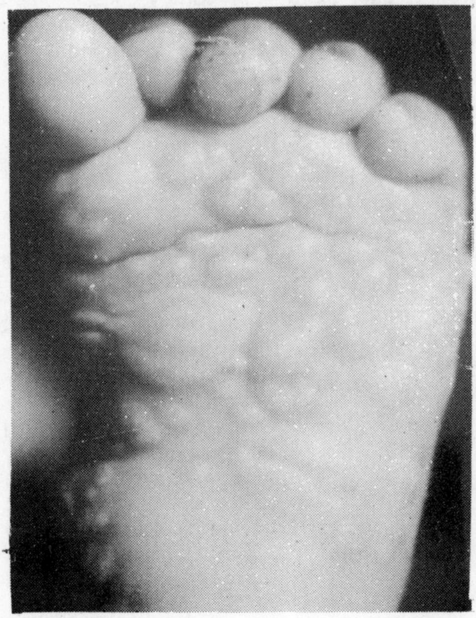

**Fig. 13. Extensive pustulations on the sole of feet of one month old infant, as an allergic reactions to scabies. Congenital syphilis used to show vesicle an palms and soles in the past but now is unusual**

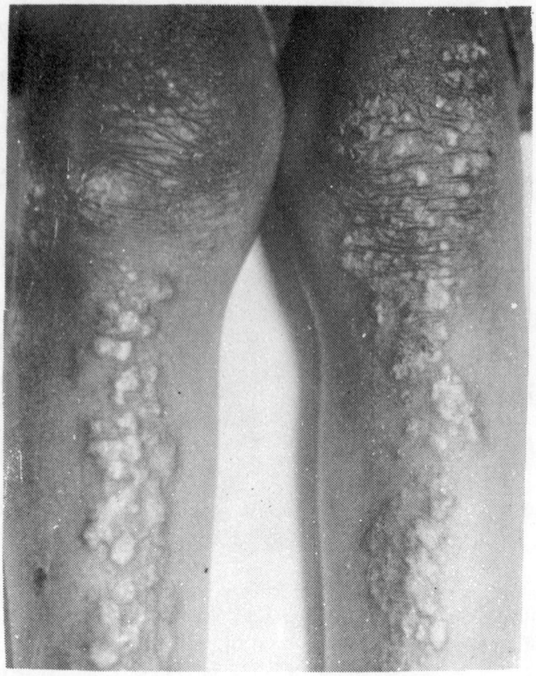

Fig. 14. Epidermolysis bullosa with residual scars. A hereditary consolidation that make the skin develop blisters with minimal injury. Sometimes, it may be quite incapicitating. It can travel in families, but unlike AIDS is non-infective.

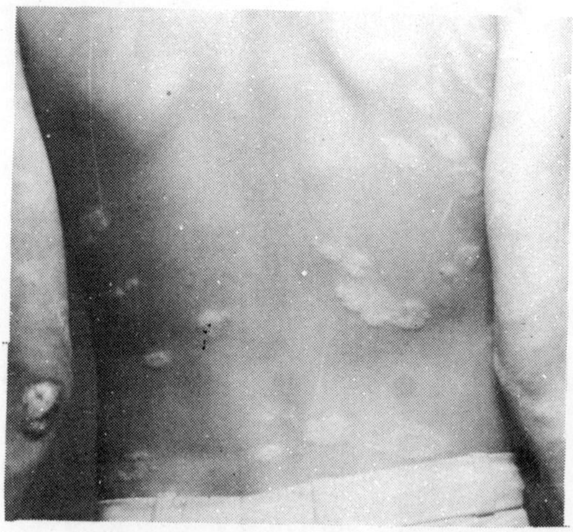

Fig. 15. A case of leprosy. The skin lesions are infiltrated patches disposed bilaterally all over the body. India being endemic for leprosy may face more difficulties due to the coexistence of the two entities. The incidence of infectious forms of leprosy may increase in AIDS.

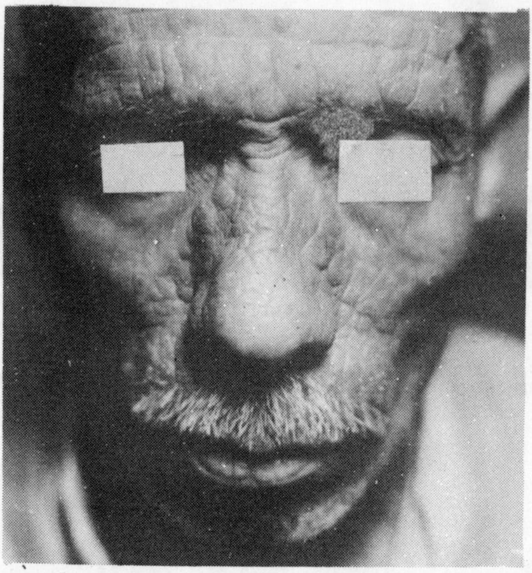

**Fig. 16. Air borne contact dermatitis. This common allergic manifestation may become an uncommon problem of AIDS patients due to a lowered cell mediated immunity.**

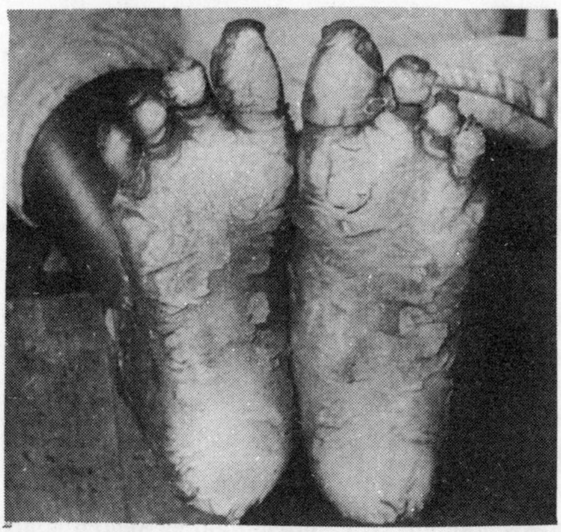

**Fig. 17. Thick keratodermic 'sandel' of Pityriasis rubra pilaris. It can also be observed in psoriasis. Its frequency in AIDS appears to be no different than in general population.**

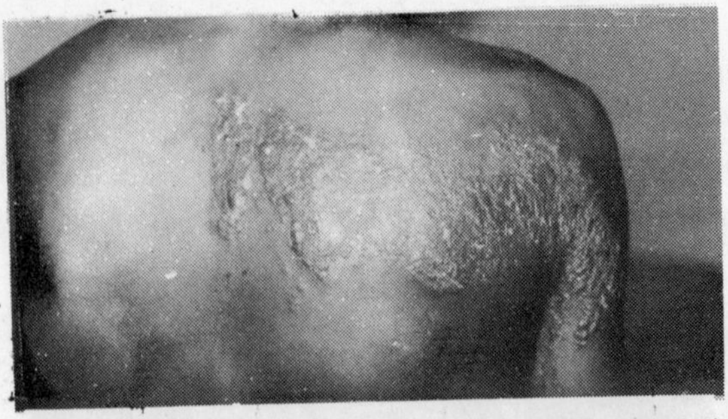

Fig. 18. Herpes zoster. The recrudescence of this chicken pox virus alongwith the dermatomes in not uncommon is AIDS. Further, the involvement of multiple dermatomes or dissimenated Herpes zoster is frequently reported in AIDS. Oral acyclovir therapy and/or prophylaxis is warranted for long periods.

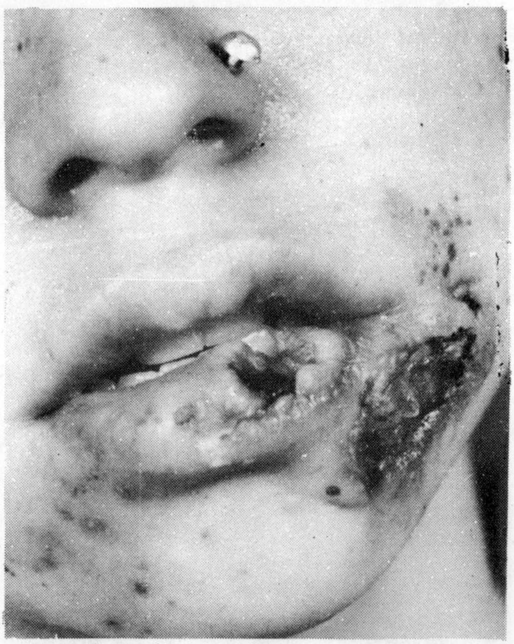

Fig. 19. Chronic myeloid leukaemia presenting as severe anaemia and bizarre ulcers on lips and face, in an 18 year old girl. The frequency of such malignancies does not seem to be increased in AIDS.

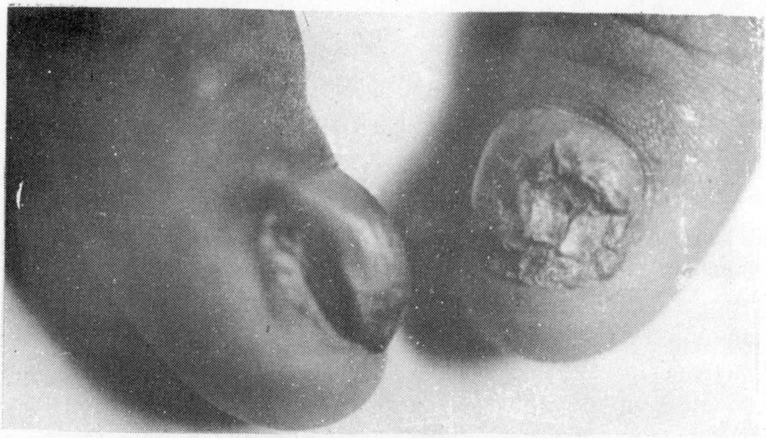

Fig. 20. Fungal infection of the nail, or for that matter any other trivial appearing bacterial, viral or fungal infection may be the first pointer to AIDS, especially if it is resistant to treatment or recurs repeatedly.

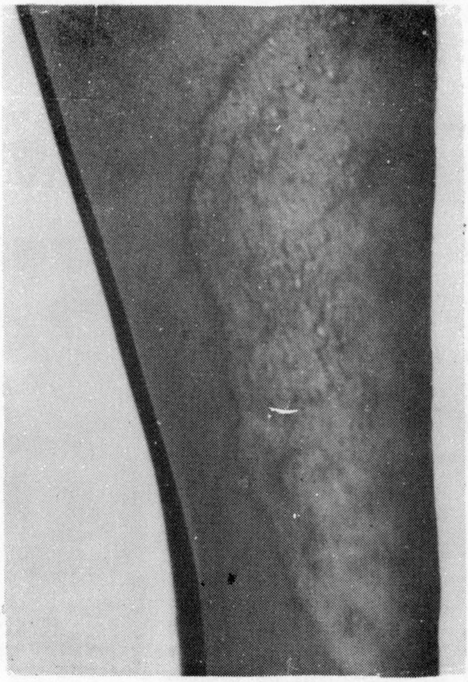

Fig. 21. Tinea incognito on the arm. Topical corticosteroids may modify the common ringworm infections, and thus continue its persistence and increase. It may erroneously be taken as some serious disease due to mistaken identity.

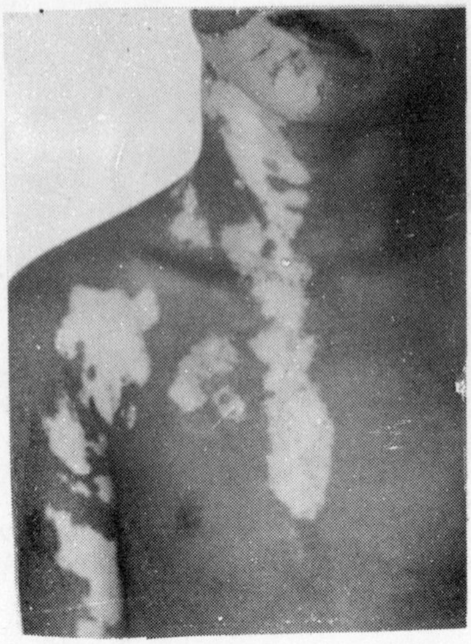

**Fig. 22. Vitiligo zosteriformis, a benign depigmenting disorder, however much it may look cosmetically disfiguring, it is non-infective and compatible with normal existence.**

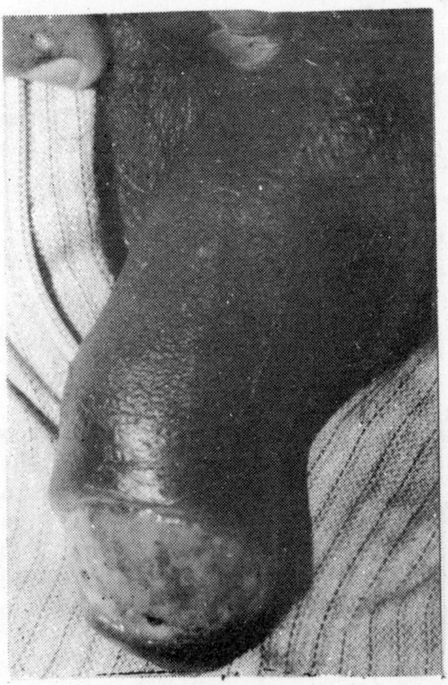

**Fig. 23. Phagedenic ulcer on the penis, a sexually transmitted disease, may point towards promiscuity, and thus increased chances of getting AIDS too.**

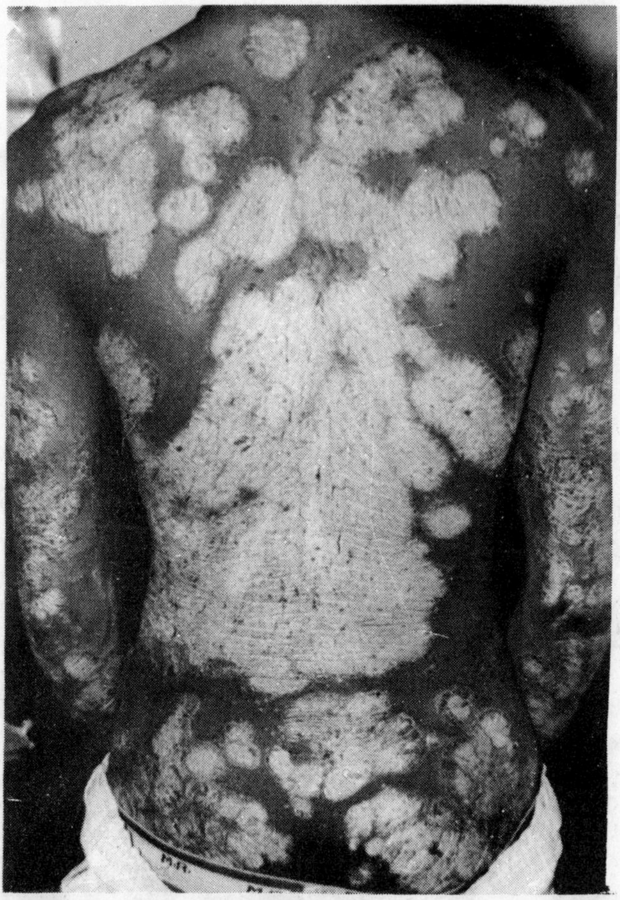

**Fig. 24.** Psoriasis vulgaris, an extensive scaling disorder with genetic predisposition and precipitation by several factors/events. It may precipitate out due to extreme stress after the diagnosis of AIDS in a susceptible individual.

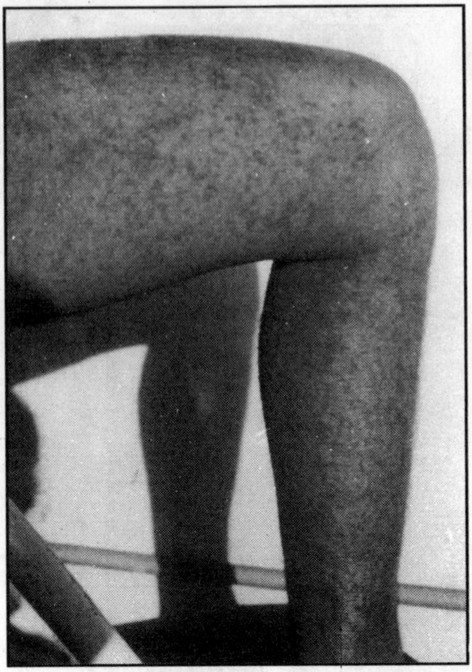

**Fig. 25. Drug-induced purpura. Drugs used for various disorders may cause depletion of platelets in the blood, thus causing wide-spread bleeding from the vessels. However, Anti-AIDS drugs rarely cause this reaction.**

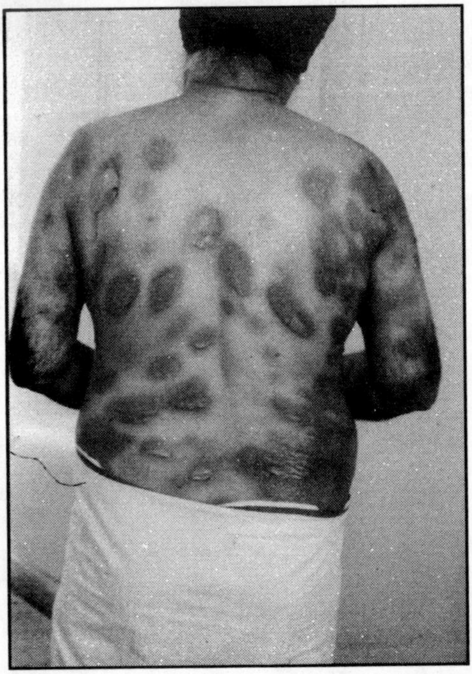

**Fig. 26. Extensive fixed drug eruption due to griseofulvin. Antiretroviral therapy is un-likely cause while therapy for opportunistic infection such as sulfa drugs may often reveal such a reaction.**

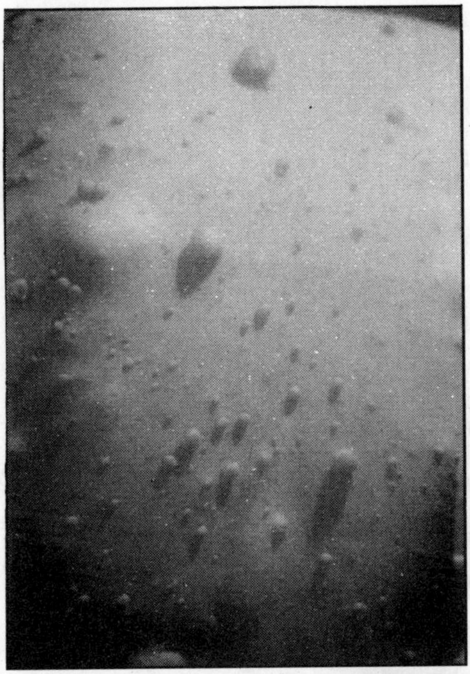

**Fig. 27. Wide-spread lesions of Neurofibromatosis on back. A hereditary disorder, transmissable to children is more cosmetic than life threatening, and has no cure.**

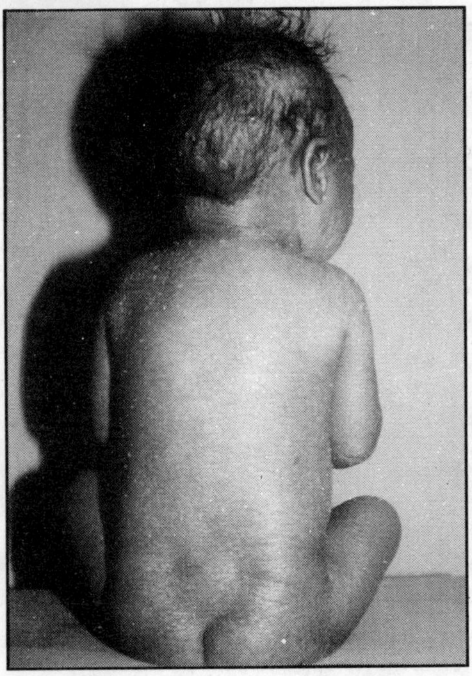

**Fig. 28. Erythroderma in a young child. It can be induced by some drug therapy. With treatment, it has recellant prognosis.**

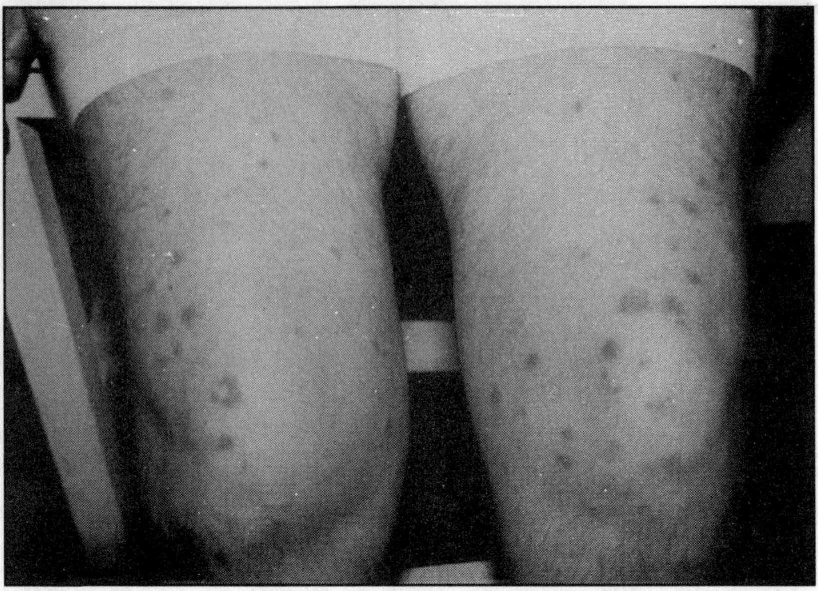

Fig. 29. Sarcoidosis. Apart from cutaneous manifestations, it also affects the body systems. A chronic disorder, it requires a prolonged multisystem therapy.

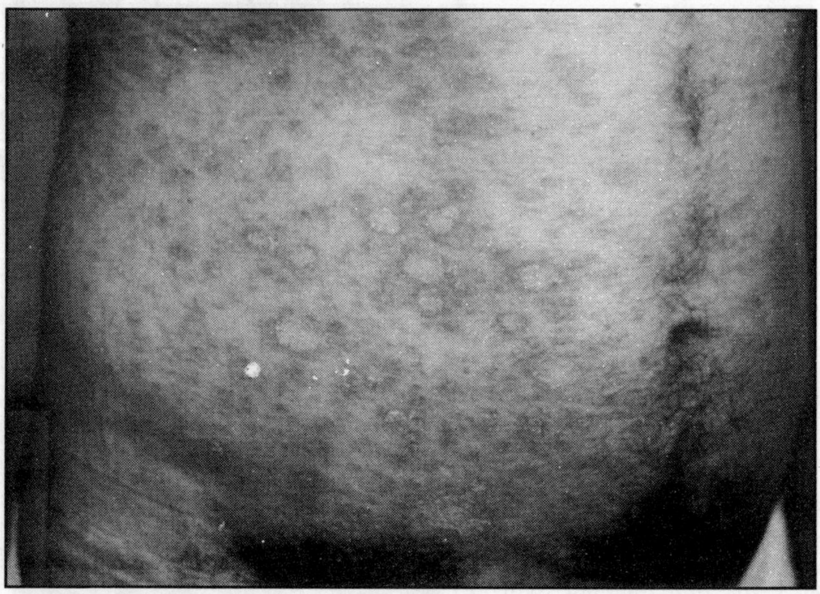

Fig. 30. Toxoallergic drug rash. It can be seen in patients of AIDS under treatment for opportunistic infections.

# Bibliography


1. Abrams DI, Lewis BH, Beckstread JH, *et al.* Persistent diffuse lymphadenopathy in homosexual men-endpoint or prodrome? *Ann Intern med* 1984; *100*: 801.
2. Abramson SD, Odajnyk CM, Grieco AJ, *et al.* Hyperalgesic pseudothromophlebtis: new syndrome in male homosexuals. *Am J Med. 1985;* 78: 317.
3. Ackerman AB. Subtle clues to diagnosis by conventional microscopy. The patch stage of Kaposi's sarcoma. *Am J Dermatopathol* 1979; *1*:165.
4. Alizon M, Wain-Hobson S, Montagnier L, *et al.* Genetic variability of AIDS-virus nucleotide analysis of two isolates. *Cell 1986; 46*:63.
5. Alonzo R, Heiman-Patterson, T, Mancall EL. Cerebral toxo-plasmosis in acquired immune deficiency syndrome. *Arch Neurol* 1984; *41*: 321.
6. Alter HJ, Eichberg JW, Maiser H, *et al.* Transmission of HTLV-III infection from donor plasma to chimpanzees: an animal model for AIDS. *Science* 1984; *226*:549.
7. Ammann AJ, Abramsa D, Contant M, *et al.* Acquired immune dysfunction in homosexual men: Immunologic profiles. *Clin Immunol Immunopathol* 1983; *27*:315.
8. Andreani T, Medigliani R, Carpentier Y, *et al.* Acquired immunodeficiency with intestinal cryposporidiosis: Possible transmission by Haitian whole blood. *Lancet* 1983; *1*:1187.
9. Anna E, Vreeburg M. Clinical observations on leprosy patients with HIV 1-infection in Zambia. *Lep Rev* (1992) 63, 134-140.
10. Anonymous. HIV and AIDS Surveillance in India. National AIDS Control programme, Ministry of Health, India 2002.
11. Balthazar EJ, Megibow AJ, Hulnick DH. Cytomegalovirus oesophagitis and gastritis in AIDS. *Am J Roentgen* 1985: *144*:1201.
12. Barbara JAJ, Contreras M, Hewitt P. AIDS: a problem for the transfusion service? *J App Med,* 1988; *14*:75.

13. Barre-sinoussi F, Chermann JC, Rey F, *et al.* Isolation of T-lymphotropiuc retrovirus from a patient at risk for acquired immunodeficiency syndrome (AIDS). *Science* 1983; 220:868.
14. Barter S. The radiology of AIDS. *J App Med*, 1988; *14*:483.
15. Barter S. Radiological features of AIDS. *Clin Immunol Allergy* 1986; *6*:601.
16. Bayley AC, Dowining RG, Cheingsong-Popov R, *et al.* HTLV-III serology distinguishes a typical and endemic Kaposi's sarcoma in Africa, *Lancet* 1985: *1*:359.
17. Beckstead JH, Wood GS, Fletcher V. Evidence for the origin of Kaposi's sarcoma from lymphatic endothelium. *Am J Pathol.* 1985; *119*:294.
18. Binford CH. Dooley JR. Aspergilliosis. *In* Binford CH, Connor DH (eds): Pathology of Tropical and Extra-ordinary Diseases, p.562. Washington, DC, Armed Forces Institute of Pathology 1976.
19. Binford CH, Dooley JR. Cryptococcosis. *In* Binford CH, Connor DH (editors), Pathology of tropical and extraordinary diseases, p. 572; Armed Force Institute of Pathology, Washington DC, 1976.
20. Binford CH, Dolley JR, Histoplasmosis. *In* Binford CH, Connor. DH (eds): Pathology of tropical and Extraordinary Diseases, p. 578. Washington, DC, Armed Forces Institute of Pathology, 1976.
21. Borton LK, Wintroub BU. Disseminated cryptococcosis presenting as herpetiform lesions in a homosexual man with acquired immuno-deficiency syndrome. *J Am Acad DErmatol.* 1984; *10*: 387.
22. Bowan DL, Lane HC, Fauci AS. Immunological features of AIDS. *In* AIDS. 1st Edition, *Pp* 89-110, *Eds* Devita Vt, Jr, Hollman S, Resenberg SA. JB Lippincott Company, Philadelphia, 1985.
23. Broder S, Gallo RC. A pathogenic retrovirus (HTLV-III) linked to AIDS, *N Engl J Med* 1984; *311*:1292.
24. Brynes RK, Chan WC, Spire TJ, *et al.* Value of lymphnode biopsy in unexplained lymphadenopathy in homosexual men. *JAMA* 1983; *250*:1313.
25. Burrage TG, Andiman WA, Katz BZ, *et al.* Virus-like rods in a lymphoid line from an infant with AIDS. *N Engl J Med* 1984; *310*:669.
26. Carrasco DA, Tyung SK. Advances in HIV treatment and treatment strategies *Med Dermatol* 2001; *19*:757-72.
27. Catania JA, Coates TJ, Stall R, *et al.* Prevalence of AIDS-related risk factors and condom use in he United States. Science 1992; *258*:1101-6.
28. CDC Division of HIV/AIDS Prevention. Basic Statistics. National Centre for HIV, STD and TB Prevention, National Institutes of Health, Washington, 2002.
29. Centers for Disease Control. Update on acquired immune deficiency syndrome (AIDS)-United States. *MMWR* 1982; *31*:507.
30. Centres for Diseases Control. Acquired Immmunodeficiency syndrome (AIDS)-Precautions for clinical and laboratory staff. *MMWR* 1982; *31*:577.

31. Centres for Disease Control. Update on acquired immunodeficiency syndrome (AIDS) among parties with hemophilia-A *MMWR*; 1982; *31*:644.
32. Centres for Disease Control. An evaluation of the acquired immunodeficiency syndrome (AIDS) reported in health-care personnel-United State. *MMWR* 1983; *32:*558.
33. Centres for Disease Control. Prevention of acquired immuno-deficiency syndrome (AIDS); Report of interagency recommendations. *MMWR* 1983; *32:*101.
34. Centres for Disease Control. Experimental infection of chimpanzees with lymphanenopathy-associated virus. *MMWR*, 1984: *33*:442.
35. Centres for Disease Control. Update-Acquired immune deficiency syndrome in persons with haemophilia. *MMWR*, 1984; *33*:589.
36. Centres for Disease Control. Update-Acquired immunodeficiency Syndrome-United States 1981-1988. *MMWR* 1989; *38*:229.
37. Centres for Disease Control. Update: acquired immunodeficiency syndrome-United States, 1991. *MMWR* 1992: *41:*463-8.
38. Centres for Disease Control. HIV instruction and selected HIV-risk behaviours among high school students-United States, 1989-1991. *MMWR* 1992; *41*:866-8.
39. Centres for Disease Control. Selected behaviours that increase risk for HIV infection, other sexually transmitted diseases, and unintended pregnancy among high school students-United States, 1991 *MMWR* 1992; *41*:945-50.
40. Centres for Disease Control. Sexual risk behaviours of STD clinic patients before and after Earvin "Magic" Johnson's HIV-infection announcement-Maryland, 1991-1992. *MMWR* 1993; *42*:45-8.
41. Centres for Disease Control. HIV/AIDS surveillance report. Atlanta: US Department of Health and Human Services, Public Health Service, May 1993: 18-9.
42. Chakrabarti S. Expression of the HTLV-III envelop gene in recombinent vaccinia viruses. *Nature* 1986; *320:*535.
43. Chanarat N, Chamarat P, Viratsetasin K *et al.* Biochemical and haematological manifestations of HIV/AIDS in Chiang Mai, Thailand. *South East Asian J. Trop Med Public Health* 2001; *32:*500-3.
44. Chernosky ME, Finley VK. Yellow nail syndrome in patients with acquired immunodeficiency disease. *J Am Acad Dermatol* 1985; *13:*731.
45. Childhood AIDS-*Pediatric clinics of North America* Paul J. Edelson M.D.-*February 1991.*
46. Christ GH, Wiener LS. Psychological issues in AIDS. *In* AIDS 1st Edition *Pp* 275-298. Eds Devita VT, Jr Hellmann S, Rosenberg SA. JB Lippincott Company, Philadelphia, 1985.
47. Church JA, Lewis J, Spotkov JM. 1gG subclass deficiencies in children with suspected AIDS. *Lancet* 1984; *1*:279.
48. Clapham, P, Weiss, R., Ralgleish A, *et al.* HIV infection of monocytes. *Virology* 1987; *149*:132.

49. Clumeck N, Sonnet J, Taelman H, *et al.* Acquired immunodeficiency syndrome in African patients. *N Engl J Med* 1984; *310*:492.
50. Coffint J, Haase A, Levij JA, *et al.* What to call the AIDS virus? *Nature* 1986; *321*:10.
51. Contreras M, Barbara J. Acquired immune deficiency syndrome and blood transfusion. *J. Hosp. Infect* 1985; *6* (Suppl. C): 27.
52. Curran JW, Lawrence DN, Jaffe H, *et al.* acquired immune deficiency syndrome associated with transfusions. *N Engl J Med* 1984; *319*:69.
53. Current WL. Human cryptosporidiosis. *N Engl J Med* 1983; *309*:1326.
54. Czelusta A, Yen-moore A, Straten MV, *et al.* An overview of sexually transmitted diseases. Part III. STDs in HIV-infected patients. *J Am Acad Dermatol* 2000:*43*: 409-32.
55. Dardenne M, Bach JF, Safai B. Low serum thymic hormone levels in patients with acquired immunodeficiency syndrome *N Engl J Med* 1983; *309*:48.
56. Dautzenberg B, Truffot C, Legris S, *et al.* Activity of clarithromycin against *Mycobacterium avium* infection in patients with the acquired immune deficiency syndrome: a controlled clinical trial. *Am Rev Respir Dis* 1992; 144:546-49.
57. Dickman S. AIDS threatens Asia. *nature 1991; 351*: 682.
58. Dictor M. Kaposi's sarcoma: origin and significance of lymphatico-venous connections. *Virchows Arch* (A). 1986; *409*: 23.
59. Diclemente RJ, Lanier MM, Horan PF, Lodico M. Comparison of AIDS attitudes and behaviours among incarcerated adolescents and a public school sample in San Francisco. *Am J Public Health* 1991; *81*:628-30.
60. Drew WL. Mintz L, Miner RC, *et al.* Prevalence of cytomegalovirus infection in homosexual men. *J Infect Dis* 1981, *143*:188.
61. Drotman DP, Curran JW. AIDS: An epidemiologic overview. *In* Friedman-Kien AE, Laubenstein LJ (eds). AIDS: The Epidemic of Kaposi's Sarcoma and Opportunistic Infections, pp 279. New York, Masson Publishing USA, 1984.
62. Eisenstat BA. Wormser GP. Seborrheic dermatitis and butterfly rash in AIDS. *N Engl J Med.* 1984; *311*:189.
63. Elie H, Laroche CA, Arnous E, *et al.* Thymic dysplasia in acquired immune deficiency syndrome. *N Engl J Med 1983;* 301:831.
64. Essex M, Hardy WD, Cotter Sw, *et al.* Naturally occuring persistent feline oncovirus infection in the absence of disease, *Infect Immunol* 1975; *11*:470.
65. Essex ME, McLane MF, Tachibana N *et al.* Seroepidemiology of himan T-cell leukaemia virus in relation to immunosuppression and acquired immunodeficiency syndrome *In* Human T-cell Leukaemia lymphoma virus. Eds Gallo RC, Essex M, Gross L. p.355. Cold Spring Harbor, 1984.
66. Ewing EP, Spira TJ, Chandler FW, *et al.* Ultrastructural markers in AIDS. *lancet* 1983; *2*:285.

67. Eving EP, Spira TJ, Chandler FW, *et al.* Unusual cytoplasmic body in lymphoid cells of homosexual men with unexplained lymphadenopathy. *N Engl J Med* 1983; *308*:819.
68. Fernandez R, Mouradian J, Metroka C, *et al.* The prognostic value of histopathology in persistent generalised lymphadenopathy in homosexual men. *N Engl J Med* 1983; *398:186.*
69. Feorino PM, Jaffe HW, Palmer E, *et al.* Transfusion associated acquired immunodeficiency syndrome. Evidence for persistent infection in blood donors. *N Engl J Med* 1986; *312*:293.
70. Finkelstein M, Berman B. HIV and AIDS in inpatient dermatology *Impatient Dermatol* 2000; *18*:509-18.
71. Fisehinger PJ, Bolognesi DP. Prospects for diagnostic tests, intervention, and vaccine development in AIDS. *In* AIDS, 1st edition *Pp 55-88*, Eds Devita VT, Jr., Hellman S. Rosenberg SA; JB Lippincott Company, Philadelphia, 1985.
72. Forgacs P, Tarshis, MA. P, *et al.* Intestinal and bronchial cryptosporidiosis in an immunodeficient homosexual man. *An Int Med* 1983; *99:*793.
73. Forthing CF, Staughton RCD, Rowland Payne CME. Skin disease in homosexual patients with acquired immune deficiency syndrome (AIDS) and lesser forms of human T cell leukaemia virus (HTLV-III) disease. *Clin Exp Dermatol,* 1985; *10*:3.
74. Francis ND, Parkin JM, Weder J, Boylston AW. Kaposi's sarcoma in acquired immune deficiency syndrome (AIDS). *J. Clin Pathol.* 1986; *39*:469.
75. Friedman-Kien AE, Lafleur FL, Gendler E, *et al.* Herpes Zoster: a possible early clinical sign for development of acquired immu-nodeficiency syndrome in high-risk individuals. *J Am Acad Dermatol.* 1986; *14*:1023.
76. Friedman AH, Freeman WR, Orellana, *et al.* Cytomegalovirus retinitis and immunodeficiency in homosexual males. *Lancet* 1982; *1*:958.
77. Friedman-Kien AE, Laubenstein LJ, Rubenstein P, *et al.* Disseminated Kaposi's sarcoma in homosexual men. *Ann Intern Med* 1982; *96*:693.
78. Gallo RC, Shaw GM, Markham PC. The etiology of AIDS. *In* AIDS. 1st Edition, Eds. DeVita VT Jr, Hellmann S, Rosenberg SA, Pp 31-54, JB Lippincott Company, Philadelphia 1985.
79. Gallo RC. Human T-cell leukaemia—lymphoma virus and T-cell malignancies in adults. *In* Franks LM, Wyke J, Weiss RA (Eds.), *Cancer Surg* 1984; *3*:113.
80. Gallo RC, Essex M Gross L (eds): Human T-Cell Leukemia Lymphoma virus, Cold Sprint Harbor NY, Cold Spring Harbor Press, 1984.
81. Gallo KC, Salahuddin SZ, Papovic M, *et al.* Frequent detection and isolation of cytopathic retrovirus (HTLV-III) from patients with AIDS, and at risk for AIDS. *Science* 1984; *224*:500.
82. Gall RC, Wong-Staal F, Sarin PS. T-cell leukemia-lymphoma virus and leukemias and lymphomas of man. *In* Goldman JM, Arrett O (eds): Mecha-

nisms of viral Leukemogensis P. 11 Edinburgh, Churchill Livingstone, 1984.

83. Gatti RA, Good RA. Occurrence of malignancy in immuno-deficiency disease. A literature review. *Cancer* 1971; *28*:89.
84. Geobert JJ, Blattner WA. The epidemiology of AIDS and related conditions, In AIDS, Ist Ed. Eds. DeVita VT, Hellman S and Rosenberg SA. *Pp* 1-30, JB Lippincott, Company, Philadelphia, 1985.
85. Goldmeier D, Psychosocial aspects of AIDS. *J App Med* 1988; *14*:91.
86. Gottlieb MS, Schroff R. Schanker HM, *et al.* Pneumocystis carinii Pneumonia and mucosal candidiasis in previously healthy homosexual men. Evidence of a new acquired immunodeficiency. *N Engl J. Med* 1981; *305*:1425.
87. Graham EJ, Rodwell MD, Toby A, *et al.* Fat redistribution in HIV Disease. *J Am Acad Dermatol* 2000; *42*:727-30.
88. Greenspan D, Greenspan JS, Conant M, *et al.* Oral 'hairy' leukoplakia in male homosexuals: evidence of association with both papillomavirus and a herpes-group virus. *Lancet*. 1984; *2*:831.
89. Green JB Sidhu GS, Lewis S, *et al. Mycobacterium avium-intercellulare*: a cause of disseminated life-threatening infection in homosexuals and drug-abusers. *Ann Intern Med* 1984; *100*:671.
90. Groopman JE, Slahuddin SZ, Sargadharan MG, *et al:* HTLV-III in saliva of people with AIDS -related complex and healthy homosexual men at risk for AIDS. *Science* 1984; *226:*337.
91. Guarda LA. Lima MA, Smith JL, Jr, *et al.* Acquired immuno-deficiency syndrome – Post mortem findings. *Am J Clin Pathol* 1984; *81*:549.
92. Guarda, LG, Silva EG, Ordonez NG, *et al.* Factor VIII in Kaposi's sarcoma. *Am J Clin Pathol* 1981; *76:*197.
93. Gyorkey F, Sinkovies JG, Gyorkey P. Tubulo-reticular structures in Kaposi's sarcoma, *Lancet* 1982; *2*:984.
94. Harris C, Small CB, Klein KS. *et al.* Immunodeficiency in female sexual partners of men with the acquired immune deficiency syndrome *N Engl J Med* 1983; *308*:181.
95. Haseltine WA, Sodroski J, Ptarca R, *et al.* Structure of 3' terminal region of type III human T lymphotropic virus: Evidence for new coding region. *Science* 1984; *225*:419.
96. Haverkos HW, Pinsky PF, Drotmon P, *et al.* Disease manifestation among homosexual men with acquired immunodeficiency syndrome: a possible role of nitrites in Kaposi's sarcoma. *Sex Transm Dis.* 1985; *12*:203.
97. Hawley DA, Schaefer JF, Schelz DM, *et al:* Cytomegalovirus encephalitis in acquired immunodeficiency syndrome. *Am J Clin Pathol* 1983; *80*:874.
98. Hochberg FA, Miller G, Schoolay RT, *et al.* Central nervous system lymphoma related to Epstein-Barr Virus. *N Engl J Med* 1983; *309*:745.
99. Hopwell PC, Luce JM: Pulmonary manifestations of the acquired immunodeficiency syndrome. *Clin Immunol Allergy* 1986; *6*:489.

100. Hruza Gj, Friedman-Kien AE, Laubenstein LJ, *et al.* Dapsone for AIDS – associated Kaposi's sarcoma, *Lancet.* 1985; *1*:642.
101. Hui AN, Koss MN, meyer PR. Necropsy findings in acquired immunodeficiency syndrome. *Hum Pathol* 1984; *15*:670.
102. Ioachim HL, Lerner CW, Tapper ML. Lymphadenopathies in homosexual men. *JAMA* 1983; *250*:1306.
103. James WD, Redfield RR, Lupton GP, *et al.* A papular eruption associated with human T cell lymphotropic virus type III disease. *J Am Acad Dermatol* 1985; *13*:563.
104. Janssen RS, Saykin AJ, Kaplan JE, *et al.* Report of International Meetings on AIDS, Paris, P 45; 1986.
105. Janier M, Vignon MD, Cottenot F. Spontaneously healing Kaposi' sarcoma in AIDS. *N Engl J Med* 1985; *312*:1638.
106. Jerrett O. Pathogenesis of feline leukaemia virus-related diseases. *In* Gldman JM, Jarrett O (eds): Mechanisms of Viral Leukemo-genesis, P 135 London, Churchill Livingstone, 1984.
107. Joachim H< Levner CW, Tapper ML. Lymphadenopathies in homosexual men – relationship with acquired immune deficiency syndrome. *JAMA* 1983: *250*:1306.
108. Jones FG, Cohen KL, Batts DH, *et al.* Disseminated histoplasmosis, invasive pulmonary aspergillosis and other opportunistic infections in a homosexual patient with acquired immune deficiency syndrome. *Sex Trnaum Dis* 1983; *10*:202.
109. Kalb RE, Grossman ME, Chronic perianal herpes simplex in immunocompromised hosts, *Am J Med* 1986; *80*:486.
110. Karon JM, Devine OJ, Morgan WM, Predicting AIDS incidence by extrapolating from recent trends. In: Castielo-Chavez C, ed. Mathe-matical and statistical approaches to AIDS epidemiology: lecture notes in biomathematics. Vol. 83. Berlin: Springer-Verlag, 1989.
111. Kennedy R, Henkel R, Paulette D, *et al.* Antiserum to a synthetic peptide recognises the HTLV-III envelop glycoprotein. *Science* 1986; *231*:1556.
112. Killen J. AIDS-related complex: a definition, *AIDS memorandum* 1984; *1*:4.
113. Kingston ME, Mackey D. Skin clues in the diagnosis of life threatening infections. *Rec infect Dis* 1986; *8*:1.
114. Kirby HB, Kenamore B, Guckian JC. *Pneumocytis carinii* pneumonia treated with pyrimethamine and sulfadiazine, *Ann Intern Med* 1971; *75*:505.
115. Klatt EC. Pathology of AIDS Version 11, Florida State University, College of Medicine, Florida, 2002.
116. Klatzmann D, Montagnier L. Approaches to AIDS therapy. *Nature* 1986; *319*:10.
117. Klein RS, Harrise CA, Small CB, *et al.* Oral candidiasis in high-risk patients as the initial manifestation of the acquired immune deficiency syndrome. *N Engl J Med* 1984; *311*:354.

118. Kotler DP, Nutritional support in AIDS. *Am J Gastroenterol 1991*; 86(5): 539-541.
119. Kreiss JK, Lawrence DN. Kasper CK, *et al.* Antibody to human T-cell leukemia virus membrane antigens, B microglobulin levels and thymosin levels in hemophiliacs and their spouses. *Ann Intern Med* 1984; *100*:178.
120. Krigel RL, Friedman-Kien AE. Kaposi's sarcoma, *In* Provost TT, Farmer ER (eds) Current Therapy in Dermatology. New York, BC Decker, 1985.
121. Kriel RL, Laubenstein LJ, Muggia FM. Kaposi's sarcoma: A new staging classification. *Cancer Treat Rep* 1983; *67*:531.
122. Krigel RL, Odajnyk CM Laubenstein LJ, *et al.* Therapeutic trial of interferon – y in patients with epidemic Kaposi's sarcoma. *J Biol response Med* 1985; *4*:358.
123. Krigel RL, Friedman-Kien AE. Kaposi's Sarcoma in AIDS. *In* AIDS Ist edition; Pp 185-212, Eds Devita VT; Jr, Hellman, S, Rosenberg SA. JB Lippincott - Raven, Philadelphia, 1997.
124. Lane HC, Masur H, Longo DL, *et al.* Partial Immune reconstitution in a patient with the acquired immunodeficiency syndrome. *N Engl Med* 1984; *311*:1099.
125. Lasky L, Berman M, Groopman J, *et al.* Neutralisation of the HIV by antibodies to a recombinant envelop glycoprotein. *Science* 1986; *233*:209.
126. Laubenstein LJ, Krigel RL, Odajnyk CM, *et al.* Treatment of epidemic Kaposi's sarcoma with etoposide or a combination of doxorubicin, bleomycin, and vinblastine. *J Clin Oncol* 1984; *2*:1115.
127. Laubenstein LJ. Staging and treatment of Kaposi's sarcoma in patients with AIDS. *In* Friedman-Kien AE, Laubenstein LJ (eds); AIDS; The Epidemic of Kaposi's Sarcoma and Opportunistic Infections, p 51. New York, Masson Publishing USA, 1984.
128. Levine AM, Meyer PR, Begandy MK, *et al.* Development of B-Cell lymphoma in homosexual men. *Ann Intern Med* 1984; *100*:707.
129. Lind SE, Gross PL, Ardiman WA, *et al.* Malignant lymphoma presenting as Kaposi's sarcoma in a homosexual man with acquired immunodeficiency syndrome. *Ann Intern Med* 1985; *102*:238.
130. Loeweinstein RJ, Sharpstein SS. Neuropsychiatric aspect of acquired immune deficiency syndrome. *Int J Psychiat Med* 1984; *13*:255.
131. Lotze MT. Treatment of immunologic disorders in AIDS. *In* AIDS, 1st Edition Pp 235-264, Ed DeVita VT, Jr, Hellman, S, Rosenberg SA. JB Lippincott - Raven, Philadelphia, 1997.
132. Louie S, Daoust PR. Schwartz RA. Immunodeficiency and Patho-genesis of non-Hodgkins lymphomas. *Semin Oncol* 1980; *7*:267.
133. Lutzner MA: Molluscum contagiosum, verruca and zoster viruses. *Arch Dermatol* 1963; *87*:436.
134. Malcolm JA, Sutherland DC. HIV and nutrition. *Lancet 1991;* 338-760.
135. Mangkornkanok-Mark M, Mark AS, Donk J. Immunoperoxidase evaluation of lymphnodes from acquired immune deficiency patients. *Clin Exp Immunol* 1984; *55*:581.

136. Marx PA Maul DH, Osborn KG, *et al.* Simian AIDS – Isolation of a type-D retrovirus and transmission of disease. *Science* 1984; *223:*1083.
137. Masur H, Michelis MA, Greene JB, *et al.* An outbreak of community – acquired *Pneumocystis carinii* pneumonia. Initial manifestation of cellular immune dysfunction. *N Engl J Med* 1981; *305:*1431.
138. Masur A, Kovacs JA, Orgnibone F, Shelhamerr J, Parrillo JE. Infections complications of AIDS. *In* AIDS, 1st Edition, Pp 161-184. Editors DeVita VT, Jr, Hellman S, Rosenberg SA, JB Lippincott - Raven, Philadelphia.
139. Mathes BM, Douglass MC. Seborrheic dermatitis in patients with acquired immunodeficiency syndrome. *J Am Acad Dermatol* 1985; *13:*947.
140. Mayoral F. Penneys NS. Disseminated histoplamosis presenting as a transepidermal elimination disorder in an AIDS victim. *J Am Acad Dermatol* 1985; *13*:842.
141. McAleer WJ, Buyank EB, Maigetter RZ, *et al.* High prevalence of lymphdenopathy virus (LAV) in European hemophiliacs. *Lancet* 1984; *2*:40.
142. Metroka CE Cunningham – Rundles S, Pollock MS *et al.* Generalised lymphadenopathy in homosexual men. *Ann Intern Med* 1983; *99:*585.
143. Miller Jr, Barrett RE, Britton CB, *et al.* Progressive multifocal leukoencephalopathy in a male homosexual with T-cell immune deficiency. *N Engl J Med* 1982; *307:*1436.
144. Miller R, Bor R. AIDS: a guide to clinical counselling 2nd ed. Philadelphia: *Science Press, 1991.*
145. Miller S, Rogers JF, Ultrastructure of AIDS lympnodes. *N Engl J Med* 1983; *309:*1188.
146. Mintzer DM, REal FX, Jovino L. *et al.* Treatment of Kaposi's sarcoma and thrombocytopenia with vincristine in patients with the acquired immunodeficiency syndrome. *Ann Intern Med.* 1985; *102:*200.
147. Mirmirani P, Hessol NA, Maurer TA, *et al.* Prevalence and predictors of skin disease in the Women's Interagency HIV study (WIHS) *J Am Acad Dermatol* 2001; *44*:785-8.
148. Modlin RL, Meyer PR, Hofman FM, *et al.* T-lymphocyte subsets in lympnodes from homosexual men. *JAMA* 1983; *250*:1302.
149. Montagnier L, Grust J, Chamaret S, *et al.* Adaptation of lymphadenopathy-associated virus (LAV) to replication in EVB-transformed, B-lymphoblastoid cells lines. *Science* 1984; *225:*63.
150. Morris L, Distenfeld A, Amorosi E *et al.* Autoimmune thrombo-cytopenic purpura in homosexual men. *Ann Intern Med* 1982; *96*:714.
151. Mortimer PP, Parry JV, Mortimer JY. Which anti-HTLV-III/LAV assays for screening and confirmatory tests? *Lancet* 1985; *3*:873.
152. Moskowitz L, Hensley GT, Chan JC, *et al.* Immediate causes of death in acquired immunodeficiency syndrome. *Arch Pathol Lab Med* 1985; *109*:735.
153. Moskowitz LB, Hensley GT, Chan JC, *et al.* Brain biopsies in patients with acquired immune deficiency syndrome. *Arch Pathol Lab Med* 1984, *108:*368.

154. Muggia FM. Treatment of classical Kaposi's sarcoma: A new look. *In* Friedman-Kien AE. Laubenstein LJ (eds); AIDS: The Epidemic of Kaposi's Sarcoma and Opportunistic Infections, p 57, New York, Hasson Publishing USA, 1984.

155. Murray HW, Rubin. By, Masur H, *et al.* Impaired cell-mediated immune responses in the acquired immune deficiency syndrome: Patients with opportunistic infection fail tsecrete acivating lymphokine and gamma interferon. *n Engl J med* 1984. *310:*883.

156. Navia BA, Price RW. Central and Peripheral nervous system complications of AIDS. *Clin Immunol Allergy* 1996; *6*:543.

157. Navia BA, Jordan BD, Price RW. The AIDS dementia Complex I: Clinical features, *Ann Neurol* 1986; *19*:517.

158. NcNutt NS, Fletcher V, Conant MA. Early lesions of Kaposi's sarcoma in homosexual men: An ultrastructural comparison with other vascular proliferations in skin. *Am J Pathol* 1983; *111*:62.

159. Negelkarke NJ, Jha P, Vlas SJ, *et al.* Modelling HIV/AIDS epidemic in Botswana and India: Impact of intervention to prevent transmission *Bull world Health Org* 2002; *80*:89-96,

160. Nicols SE, Jr, Psychiatric aspects of AIDS. *Psychosomatics* 1983, *24*:1083.

161. Nwanyanwu OC, Conti L, Cielsielki Ca, *et al.* Increasing frequency of heterosexually transmitted AIDS in southern Florida: artifact or reality? *Am J Public Health* 1993; *83*:571-3. Odajnyk C, Laubenstein L. Friedman-Kien AF, *et al.*

162. Therapeutic trial of human gamma interferon (IFN) in Patients with epidemic Kaposi's sarcoma (EKS) (abstr). *Proc Am Soc Clin Oncol* 1984; *13*:61.

163. Ognibene FP, Steis RG, Machar AM, *et al.* Kaposi's sarcoma causing pulmonary infiltrates and respiratory failure in the acquired immunodeficiency syndrome. *Ann Intern Med* 1985; *102;* 471.

164. Oleske JM, Minnefor AB. Immune deficiency syndrome in children. *JAMA* 1983; *250:*3046.

165. Orenstein JM. Ultrastructural markers in AIDS. *Lancet* 1983; *2*:284.

166. Oroszlan S, Sarngadharan MG, Gallio RC, *et al.* Primary structure analysis of the major internal protein p 24 of human type C T-cell leukemia virus. *Proc. Natl Acad Sci USA* 1982; *79*:1291.

167. Pancharoen C, Thisyakorn U Pediatric acquired immunodeficiency syndrome in Asia: Mother to child transmission. *Clin Infect Dis* 2002, *34*:565-9.

168. Papovic M, Flomenberg N, Volkman DJ, *et al.* Alteration of T-cell functions by infection with HTLV-I or HTVL-II. *Science* 1984; *226*:459.1

169. Pasternak J, Boliver R, Histoplasmosis in acquired immuno-deficiency syndrome: diagnosis by bone marrow examination. *Arch Intern Med* 1983; *143*:2024.

170. Penn I, Depressed immunity and the development of cancer. *Clin Exp Immunol* 1981; *46*:459.

171. Penneys WS. Skin Manifestations of I AIDS, Dunitz, London 1990.
172. Pinching AJ. Review: The acquired immune deficiency syndrome. *Clin Exp Immunol* 1984: *56*:1.
173. Pitchenik AE, Rubinson HA. The radiographic appearance of tuberculosis in patients with acquired immunodeficiency syndrome (AIDS) and pre-AIDS. *Am Rev Resp Dis.,* 1985: *131*:393.
174. Pitchenik AE, Fischl MA. Disseminated tuberculosis and the acquired immunodeficiency syndrome. *Ann Intern Med.* 1983; *98*:112.
175. Poiesz BJ, Ruscetti FW, Reitz MS, *et al.* Isolation of a new type C retrovirus (HTLV) in primary uncultured cells of a patient with Sezary T-cell leukaemia. *Nature* 1981; *294*:268.
176. Polski B, Gold JWM, Whimbey E, *et al.* Bacterial pneumonias in patient with the acquired immunodeficiency syndrome. *Ann Intern Med* 1986; *504*:38.
177. Prince HE, Gottlieb MS, Kermani-Arab V, *et al.* Interleukin-2 receptor: Relationship to defective T-cell proliferation in acquired immune deficiency syndrome. *Fed Proc* 1983; *42*:1334.
178. Prince HE, Karmani-Arab V, Fahey JL: Depressed interleukin-2 receptor expression in acquired immune deficiency syndrome and lymphadenopathy syndromes. *J Immunol* 1984; *133*:1313.
179. Quinnan GV, Masur H, Rook AH, *et al.,* Herpes virus infections in the acquired immunodeficiency syndrome, *JAMA* 1984; *252*:72.
180. Rampen FHJ. AIDS and the dermatologist. *Int J. Dermatol* 1987; *26*:1.
181. Rao TKS, Filippone EJ, Nicastri AD, *et al.* Associated focal and segmental glomerulosclerosis in the acquired immune deficiency syndrome, *N Engl J Med* 1984; *310*:669.
182. Rapp F. Cytomegalovirus and carcinogenesis. *J Natl Cancer Inst* 1984; *72*:783.
183. Ratner L, Haseltine W, Patarca R, *et al.* Complete nucleotide sequence of the AIDS Virus, HTLV-III. *Nature* 1985; *313*:277.
184. Redfield RR, James WD, Wright DC, *et al.* Severe molluscum contagiosum infection in a patient with human T-cell lymphotropic (HTLV-III) disease. *J Am Acad Dermatol* 1985; *13*:821.
185. Reichert CM, O'Leary TJ, Levens DL, *et al.* Autopsy pathology in the acquired immune deficiency syndrome. *Am J Pathol* 1983; *122*:357.
186. Reichert CM, Kelly VL, Macher AM. Pathologic features of AIDS. *In* AIDS 1st Edition *Pp* 111-160, Ed DeVita VT, Jr. Hellaman S, Rosenberg SA, JB Lippincott Company, Philadelphia 1985.
187. Robert-Guroof M, Safai B, Glemann E, *et al.* HTLV-I specific antibody in AIDS patients and others at risk. *Lancet* 1984; *2*:128.
188. Robert-Guroff M, DGallo RC. Establishment of an etiologic relationship between the human T-cell leukemia/lymphoma virus (HTLV) and adult T-cell leukemia. *Bulletin* 1983; *1*:45.
189. Rook AH, Masur H, Lane HC, *et al.* Interleukin 2 enhances the depressed

natural killer and cytomegalovirus-specific cytotoxic activities of lymphocytes from patients with the acquired immune deficiency syndrome. *J Clin Invest* 1983; *72*:398.

190. Rotterdam H, Lerner CW, Tapper ML. Biopsies of the digestive tract in patients with acquired immunodeficiency syndrome. *Lab Invest* 1983; *48*:72.
191. Rubenstein A, Sicklick M, Gupta A, *et al.* Acquired immuno-deficiency with reversed T4/T8 ratios in infants born to promiscuous and drug-addicted mother. *JAMA* 1983; *249*:2350.
192. Rustgi V, Hoofnagle J, Gerin J, *et al.* Hepatitis B viral infection in patients with the AIDS. *Ann Intern Med* 1984; *101*:795.
193. Rustgers JL, Wieczorek R: Bonetti F, *et al.* The expression of endothelial cell surface antigens by AIDS-associated Kaposi's sarcoma. *Am J Pathol* 1986; *122*:493.
194. Safai B, Groopman Je, Popovic M, *et al.* Seroepidemiological studies of human T-lymphotropic retrovirus type III in acquired immunodeficiency syndrome. *Lancet* 1984; *1*:1438.
195. Safai B, Koziner B. Malignant neoplasma in AIDS. *In* AIDS, Ist Ed. *Pp* 231-222, Eds DeVita VT, Jr, Hellman S, Rosenberg SA, JB Lippincott Company, Philadelphia, 1985.
196. Salahuduin SZ, Karkham PD, Lindner SG, *et al.* Lympholine production by cultural human T-cell transformed by human T-cell leukemia-lymphoma virus. *Science* 1984; *223*:703.
197. Sarngadharan MG, Popovič M, Bruch L, *et al.* Antibodies reactive with human T-lymphotropic retroviruses (HTLV-III) in the serum of patients with AIDS. *Science* 1984; *243*:506.
198. Schwartz JL, Muhlbauer JE, Steigbigel RT. Pre-Kaposi's sarcoma, *J Am Acad Dermatol*, 1984; *11*:377.
199. Schubach J, Popovic M, Giledn RV, *et al.* Serological analysis of human T-lymphotropic retroviruses (HTLV-III) associated with AIDS. *Science* 1984; *224*:503.
200. Shaw GM, Hahn BH, Arya BK, *et al.* Molecular characterisation of HTLV-III in AIDS. *Science* 1984; *226*:1165.
201. Shaw GM, Hahn BH, Popovic M, *et al.* Molecular cloning and analysis of different human T-lymphotropic retroviruses from patients with AIDS or T-cell malignancy. *In* Gottlieb MJ, Groopman JE (eds): Acquired Immune Deficiency Syndrome. UCLA Symposium on Molecular and Callular Biology, Vol. 16, p. 59. New York, Alan R Liss, 1984.
202. Sidhu GS. Stahl RE, El-Sadr W, *et al.* Ultrastructural markers of AIDS. *Lancet* 1983; *1*:990.
203. Siegal FP. Normal delayed-type skin reactions in early stages of acquired cellular immunodeficiency. *N Engl J Med* 1982; *307*:184.
204. Siegal FP. Immune functions and dysfunctions in AIDS. *Semin Oncol* 1984; *11*:29.

205. Simmons BP, Hooton TM, Mallison GF. Guidelines for hospital environmental control. *Infect Control* 1981 *2:*131.
206. Skis R, Broder S. AIDS: A general overview. *In* AIDS, Ist Ed. *Pp* 299-338 Eds. DeVita VT, Jr., Hellmann S, Rosenberg SA JB Lippincott Company Philadelphia, 1985.
207. Snider WO, Simpson DM, Nielson T, *et al.* Neurological compli-cations of acquired immune deficiency syndrome. Analysis of 50 patients. *Ann Neurol* 1983; *14:*403.
208. Sodroski J. Goh W, Rosen C, *et al.* REplicative and cytopathic potential of HIV with Sor gene deletions. *Science* 1986; *23:*1549.
209. Soeprono PF, Schinella RA, Cockerell CJ, Comite SL. Seboreeheic-like dermatitis of acquired immunodeficiency syndrome; a clinico-pathologic study. *J Am Acad Dermatol* 1986; *14:*242.
210. Soeprono FF, Schinella RA. Eosinophilic pustular folliculitis in patients with acquired immunodeficiency syndrome; report of three cases. *J Am Acad Dermatol* 1986; *14:*1020.
211. Spach D, Kein P, Human Immunodeficiency virus and the acquired immunodeficiency syndrome. *In* Altas of STDs and AIDS IInd Ed, Eds Morse SA *et al.* Mosby-Wolfe, Philadelphia, 1996.
212. Special report. Infection control guidelines for patients with the acquired immunodeficiency syndrome (AIDS). *N Engl J Med* 1983; *309:*740.
213. Spira TJ, Des Jarlais DC, Marmor M, *et al:* Prevalence of antibody to lymphadenopathy-associated virus among drug-detoxification patients in New York. *n Engl J Med* 1984; *468:*48.
214. Storm RL, Gruninger RP. AIDS with *Mycobacterium avium-intercellulare* lesions resembling those of Whipple's disease. *N Engl J Med* 1983; *309:*1323.
215. Szmuness W, Much I, Prince AM. *et al.* On the role of sexual behaviours in the spread of hepatitis B infection, *Ann Intern med* 1975; *83:*849.
216. Vass AA. AIDS – a plague in us. Venue Academica. St. Ives, Cambridge, 1986.
217. Volberding P, Moran T, Abrams D, *et al.* Recombinant alpha interferon (aIFN) therapy of Kaposi's sarcoma (KS) in the acquired immune deficiency syndrome (AIDS). *Blood* 1983; *62* Supple 1):118.
218. Volberding P, Kaslow K, Bille M, *et al:* Prognostic factors in staging Kaposi's sarcoma in the acquired immune deficiency syndrome (abstr). *Proc Am Soc Clin Oncol* 1984; *3:*51.
219. Wain Hobson S, Sonigo P, Danos O. Nucleotide sequence of the AIDS virus, LAV. *Cell* 1985; *40:*9.
220. Warner LC, Fisher BK. Cutaneous manifestations of the acquired immunodeficiency syndrome. *Int J Dermatol.* 1986; *25:*337.
221. Weber JN, Roger LA, Scott K, *et al.* Three-year prospective study of HTLV-III/LAV infection in homosexual men. *Lancet* 1986; *1:*1179.
222. Wober J. AIDS: The virus, antivirals and vaccines. *J App Med* 1988; *14*:81.

223. Whang-peng J, Lee EC, Sieverts H. *et al.* Burkitt's lymphoma in AIDS; Cytogenetic study. *Blood* 1984; *6 4:*818.
224. Whelan MA, Kricheff II, Handler M, *et al.* Acquired immunodeficiency syndrome; Cerebral computed tomographic manifestations. *Radiology* 1983; *149*:477.
225. Wong G, Gold JWM, Brown AE, *et al.* Central nervous system toxoplasmosis in homosexual men and parentral drug abusers. *Ann Intern Med* 1984; *100:*34.
226. Wright K. AIDS therapy. *Nature* 1986; *232:*283.
227. Yoshida M, Seiki M, Yamaguchi K, *et al.* Monoclonal integration of HTLV provirus in all primary tumors of adult T-cell leukemia suggests causative role of HTLV in the disease. *Proc natl Acad Sci USA* 1984; *81*:2534.
228. Young LS, Wiviott L, Wu M, Kolononski P, Bolan R, Inderlied CB. Azithromycin for treatment of *Mycobacterium avium-intracellulare* complex infection in patients with AIDS. *Lancet* 1991; *338:*1107-9.
229. Zagury D, Bernard J, Leibowitch J, *et al.* HTLV-III in cells cultured from semen of two patients with AIDS. *Science* 1984; *226*:449.
230. Ziegler JL, Beckstead JA, Volberding PA, *et al.* Non-Hodgkin's lymphoma in 90 homosexual men. *N Engl J Med* 1984; *311:*565.
231. Zolla-Pazner S, William D, El-Sadr W, *et al.* Quntitation of $B_2$-microglobulin and other immune characteristics in a prospective study of men at risk for acquired immune deficiency syndrome. *JAMA* 1984; *251:*2951.
232. DHHS Guidelines for the use of antiretroviral agents in HIV-infected adults and adolescents November, 2003.
233. WHO Guidelines for the use of antiretroviral therapy in resource-constrained countries Dec. 1, 2003.
234. AIDS Therapy Dolin R, Masur H and Saag MS, Eds. Churchill-Livingstone 2003.
235. Reiter G.S. Comprehensive Clinical Care: Managing HIV as a chronic illness, AIDS Clinical Care February 2000; 12(2): 13-19
236. Manual of HIV Therapeutics. Powderly WG, Ed. Lippincott Williams and Wilkins 2001.
237. The AID Knowledge Base Cohen PT, Sande MA and Volberding PA, Eds. Lippincott Williams and Wilkins 1999.
238. Yeni P.G., Hammer S.M., Saag MS *etal* Treatment of adult HIV infection 2004 recommendations of the International AIDS Society-USA Panel. JAMA, 2004; 292: 251-265.

# Index


Abacavir 120, 123
Acquired immunodeficiency
  syndrome (AIDS)
  acute infection 31-33
  childhood AIDS 17, 46-47
  chimpanzee model 18, 38
  clinical features 37-45
  cutaneous manifestations 39-43
  definition CDC 18-20
  WHO 16-17
  demography of 4-15
  diagnosis 105-114
  etiology 3, 29
  Incubation period 30, 31
  infections in 74-94
  lesser-AIDS 37, 38
  malignancies in 97-100
  paediatric- 17, 48-56
  pathology 57-73
  prevention of 139-147
  simian- 18, 38
  therapy of 115-136
  vaccine, preparations 137-139
Acyclovir 134, 136
Adoptive immunotherapy 118-119
Africa, demography of AIDS
  in 13, 14
AIDS-related complex 17, 101-102
  clinical features 101, 102
  definition 101
  differential diagnosis 103
  follow up 103
  histopathology 103
Alpha interferon 116, 117, 136
Amphotericin-B 133, 134
Amprenavir 120, 126
Anal intercourse 22
Ansamycin, clofazimine 134
  plus, in AIDS 134
Antibodies, HTLV-III 107, 108, 111
Anti-viral agents 120, 123, 129
  site of activity 120
  comparative study 123, 129
Anti-viral antibody therapy 119
  see also immunotherapy
Aspergillosis 86, 87

B-cell dysfunctions 72
Bacillary angiomatosis 41, 42
bacterial infections 89-92, 127, 129
Blood product recipients 24
Body piercing 164
Breast feeding 159
Butterfly eruptions 41

Candidiasis 84, 133
$CD_4$+ cells 9, 10, 70-71, 107
$CD_8$ cells 9, 10, 70-71, 108
Chemotherapy of Kaposi's
  sarcoma 115-135
Children of AIDS patients 3, 4
Cimetidine 118

Coccidioiodomycosis 86, 87
Combivir 120
Condyloma acuminata 89
Cryptococcosis 16, 17, 85, 133
Cryptosporidiosis 17, 83, 84
Cutaneous anergy 43, 46
Cytomegalovirus (CMV)
    infection 17, 86, 87, 134
    Kaposi's sarcoma, and 86
    Retinochorioditis 88, 89
    Treatment of 134, 135

Definition, AIDS 16-20
    AIDS-related complex 17, 101, 102
    lesser AIDS 18
    Paediatric AIDS 18, 46
    persistent generalised
    lymphodenopathy (PGL) 18-20
    Simian AIDS 18
Demography of AIDS, 4-14
    Africa 12, 13
    Europe 13
    Global 3, 4
    Haiti 12, 24, 25
    India 4-8
    United States 8-12
Delavirdine 120, 124, 129
Diarrhoea 18, 79, 80
Didanosine 120, 122
Disinfection 141-144
Drug abusers, parentral 2, 23, 24

Efavirenz 120, 122
Electron microscopic
    findings 61, 68, 69, 74
Encephalitis, *Toxoplasma* 17, 83
Enzyme-linked
    immunosorbent assay
    (ELISA) 109, 110, 112
Epstein-Barr virus (EBV) 89, 90
Europe, AIDS in 13

Female partners 24-26
Fever, evaluation 76-82
Flucytosine, in
    cryptococcosis 133
Fungal infections,
    aspergillosis 86, 87
    candidiasis 17, 74, 84
    coccidioiodomycosis 86, 87
    cryptococcosis 17, 74, 85
    histoplasmosis 85, 86

Gallium scan, in
    *Pneunocystis carinii* 174
    pneumonia 74, 75
Gamma interferon 116, 117
Gastrointestinal tract
    involvement in Aids 79, 83
Gingivitis 42

Haitians 13, 24
Haemophiliacs 23
Hairy leukoplakia, oral 42, 43
Hepatitis-B infection 89, 90
Herpes simplex virus
    infection 88-89
Herpes zoster 89
Heterosexual contacts 23-25
Histoplasmosis 85-86
HIV-1 1, 3, 5, 16-17, 28-29
    Biologic properties 28, 29
    Salient features 31
HIV-Disease 38-40, 107, 111
    CDC classification 38, 39
    Diagnostic tests 110
Hodgkin's disease 13
Homosexual males 1, 19-22
HTLV-III virus, biologic
    properties 3, 28-36
    cytopathic effects 29
    isolation of 3, 24-27
    molecular biology 30, 31
    sero-epidemiology 2-4
    vaccine against 136-138
Hyperalgesic
    pseudothrombophlebitis 42, 43

Idiopathic
    thrombocytopenic purpura 101
Immunofluorescence
    HTLV-III antibodies 107-112
    HTLV-III antigens 111-113
Immunologic features, of

AIDS 70-73
AIDS-related complex 70, 71
high-risk groups 22
Immunomodulators 117-118
Immunotherapy 118, 119, 136
Inclusion bodies, test-tube
ring-shaped 68
tubuloreticular 68, 113
vesicular rosettes 68
viral-type 61, 68
India, demography of AIDS 4-8
Indinavir 120, 125
Infectious complications, 74-93
aspergillosis 86
bacterial infections 89-93
candidiasis 17, 74, 84, 133
coccidioiodomycosis 86-87
condyloma acuminata 89
cryptococcosis 16, 17, 85, 133
crytosporodiosis 17, 83
cytomegalovirus 17, 86-89
enteric pathogens 79, 91-92
Epstein-Barr virus 89, 90
fungal infections 17, 84-87
Hepatitis-B virus 89, 90
herpes simplex 88-89
herpes zoster 89
histoplasmosis 85, 86
molluscum contagiosum 89
*Mycobacterium avium-intercellulare* 17, 74-76, 133
*Mycobacterium tuberculosis*
opportunistic 17, 74, 133
*Pneumocystis carinii* 74-79
pneumonia 74-77
progressive multi-focal 76, 78
leukoencephalopathy
polyoma virus 89-90
protozoal infections 74, 79-86, 127-133
retinochoroiditis 88, 89
*Salmonella* 79, 92
Toxoplasmosis 16, 17, 74, 83-84, 133
viral infection 17, 74, 86-90
Interferons 116-117
alpha- 2, 116-117
gamma 116
Interleukin trials 116-118

Kaposi's sarcoma 1, 13, 95-99
clinical features 96-98
histopathological features 68-70, 97
staging 97
treatment 134-136
types, differentiating features 102

Lamivudine 120, 122
Lopinavir 120, 126
*Legionella* 92
Lymphadenopathy syndrome (LAS) 2, 101
Lymphadenopathy associated virus 2, 16
Lymphomas 69, 99-100

Malignancies in AIDS 14, 95-100
Mycobacterium avium-*intercellulare* 17, 74-76, 89-91, 134
*Mycobacterium tuberculosis* 17, 74, 134

Nelfinavir 120, 126, 129
Nervous system, central, 76, 78
cytomegalovirus infection 86-89
psychiatric symptoms 44, 45
psychosocial aspects 44, 46
Nevirapine 120, 124

Opportunistic infections 74-76

Paediatric AIDS 46-56
Clinical features 46-51
Diagnosis 51-56
Papulopruritic eruptions 41, 42
Pathological features of
AIDS infections 57-69, 113
Kaposi's sarcoma 68, 69
Lymphadenopathy
syndrome 58, 59
Lymphnodes 58-59
spleen 61, 68
testis 61, 68
thymus 68

Pentamidine isethionate 128, 130
Persistent generalised
lyphadenopathy 17, 19, 72
Plasmapheresis 119
*Pneumocystis carinii* 1, 9, 17, 74, 79, 84, 130
Polymerase chain reaction
Polyoma virus infection 89, 90
Pre-AIDS 70
Progressive multifocal
leukoencephalopathy 76, 78
Protozoal infections, 82-84
cryptospoidiosis 17, 83-84
*Pneumocystis carinii* 1, 9, 17, 74, 84, 185
toxoplasmosis, 16, 17, 83, 84, 133
Prurigo-like lesions 42, 43
Psychosocial issue 43-46
Psychiatric complications 43-45, 146
Pyrimethamine 132

Radioimmunoassay (RIA),
HTLV-III antibodies 108, 110
HTLV-III antigens 111-112
Radiological features 113-114
Rapid Tests
Retinitis, cytomegalovirus 88, 89
Risk factors, in Haitians 23, 24
haemophiliacs 24
heterosexual contacts 23-27
homosexual males 19-21
parentral drug abusers 23, 24
Paediatric AIDS 17, 24
transfusion recipients 23, 24
Ritonavir 120, 125

Safety precautions 139-140, 143-145
Saquinavir 120, 125
Seborrhoeic dermatitis in
AIDS 39, 41
Sexual practices in
homosexual males 19-21
Simian AIDS 18, 19, 38
Southern blotting test 112-113
Spectrum of AIDS 37-38
Splenomegaly 61, 68
State AIDS Control Societies
Stavudine 120, 122
Sterilization 141-144

Tattooing and AIDS
T-lymphocytes dysfunctions 17, 18, 70-71
lymphnodes 58, 61, 68
Thymic hormones/factors 117
*Toxoplasma gondii* 17, 18, 74, 83-84, 130
Transfusion recipient 2, 6, 23-24
Transmission of AIDS 2, 14, 18-22
perinatal transmission 24
Trizivir 120, 123

United States, demography
of AIDS 9-14

Vaccines for AIDS 137-138
prevention 138
Vasculitis, immune complex 42, 44
VCT
Vesicular rosettes 68-69
Viral infections, condyloma
acuminata 89
cytomegalovirus 17, 86-89
Epstein-Barr virus 89, 90
hepatitis-B virus 89, 90
herpes simplex 88-89
herpes zoster 89
molluscum contagiosum 89
polyoma virus 90

Walter Reed classification 107
Western electroblot test 110

Xeroderma 40-41

Yellow nail syndrome 40-41

Zalcitabine 120, 123
Zidovudine 127, 129